AN AWAKENING

How I Defeated Cancer Without Chemotherapy or Radiation

CJ Ainsworth

AN AWAKENING

How I Defeated Cancer Without Chemotherapy or Radiation

Printed in the United State of America by Createspace

ISBN 978-1522938439
ISBN 1522938435

First Edition: February 2016

10 9 8 7 6 5 4 3 2 1

Dedication

This book is dedicated first, to my husband John Ainsworth, my caregiver throughout my entire healing process. His relentless dedication helped me to achieve my healing goals throughout my two year alternative therapy program. He continues to keep me on track to ensure I have no cancer recurrence. I love him with all my heart.

I dedicate this book to Debbie Smith and Virginia Aguiles. God Bless you Virginia. Virginia was a trooper. She and Debbie Smith were my biggest supporters in writing this book. I met both of these wonderful women at The Longevity Center (TLC), a cancer healing clinic in California. They are my friends and we supported each other through our toughest ordeals. They inspired me to write my story with a cookbook to enforce the importance of proper eating and to promote a new healthy lifestyle.

Acknowledgements

I would like to thank and acknowledge our children—Matthew Stoen, Melissa Ainsworth, Jens Stoen, John Ainsworth II and Elizabeth Ainsworth—for their continuing support of my cancer treatment decision and their constant love. I would also like to thank the Gerson Therapy and Dr. Donald Stillings, DC of The Longevity Center (TLC). Thanks to all my family, especially my two sisters, Suzi Tveit Vickstrom and Julie Ann Tveit, who spent time to learn and do a part of the Gerson Therapy with me and who continually support me with my decision. Thank you to my sister in-law Patricia Proctor, who helps us feed and care for our farm animals, and thank you to all my friends, particularly Nicky Barnes, who kicks me in the butt to exercise, and to all those who continue to be there for me.

A special thanks to Deborah Inskip, our friend and nurse at Reno Integrative Medical Center and our dear friend Paul Attea who spent countless hours on the telephone guiding my husband and me through some very bad days. Thanks to David Kahn, DC, our friend and chiropractor, who assisted me along the way with his knowledge and personal experience with the Gerson Therapy and to my brother-in-law, Ronald E. Ainsworth, MD, for his allopathic (conventional) medical knowledge. Without him I would not have gone to the Stanford Cancer Center. And thanks to my editor Jennifer Skancke for her generous help and continued encouragement to complete my story and my cookbook.

Table of Contents

Introduction

This book, "An Awakening: How I Defeated Cancer without Chemotherapy or Radiation" is the story of what changed my life, breast cancer. I was horrified when I learned I had cancer and even more horrified when I was told I only had 6 months or a year to live if I did not do chemotherapy or radiation. I reveal what I went through, what I learned about breast cancer, the methods that helped me heal, and what I chose that saved me.

When we're young, most of us have dreams of how we want our lives to be. When I was young I dreamed of what it would be like when I became an adult. In my vision, I would graduate from high school, get married, and raise four boys in a beautiful home. That's what I wanted and that's what I believed would happen.

I was an athletic child. I took dancing lessons and baton lessons and became one of the drum majorettes at my high school. I started to date and was becoming popular in school. My life seemed to be unfolding.

In 1962 at 16 years old, I had an accident and fractured my lower back. I was in extreme pain and began losing my ability to walk. I went to school in a wheelchair and all my activities stopped. My doctors determined that something was damaging a nerve and they recommended back surgery. My parents were informed that the surgery was risky but there was a chance I'd be able to walk again. I had the surgery and endured months of physical therapy to walk again.

During my hospital confinement I met a young man and fell in love. In 1964, a month after I graduated from high school we were married. I was back on track with my dream. My husband's parents helped us purchase a home just a block from my parents in Fridley, Minnesota. Our home was small but perfect for young newlyweds. It had one bedroom, kitchen, living room, and a bathroom in the basement next to the boiler room. We literally had to sit on the toilet to take a shower. I laugh about it now but back then it was heaven because it was ours.

Less than a year later we discovered I was pregnant. During that time our home was damaged by a tornado. As luck would have it, my father-in-law was transferred to California. There was ample room in the moving van so we packed up what little belongings we had and moved with my in-laws leaving our home behind.

The trip was hard on me and my pregnancy was very worrisome. I was bedridden most of the term and I couldn't keep enough weight on. The doctor was concerned about my health and my ability to have a healthy baby. When my son was born he only weighed a little over 5 pounds, but he was beautiful and healthy. I named him Matthew —meaning "a gift from God." By the time I was twenty-seven, I had several miscarriages and the last one almost caused my death. I had to have a hysterectomy, another of my many health issues.

In 1972 my husband's work took him to Alaska. I was able to obtain a transfer from my job and with our young son in tow, we all moved to Alaska where my husband and his partners formed a construction company. We built a lovely home and adopted a beautiful boy, Jens. My two sons were the love of my life. The company flourished and I was able to attend college at the University of Alaska in Anchorage during the day while my boys were in school. All things were good.

By 1984 the partnership and business started to fail and eventually the company was lost. We headed back to the lower 48 and ended up in Nevada. After a long two-year legal battle with the IRS over the failed company, we declared bankruptcy. We were devastated and our marriage was also failing. After our oldest son graduated from college I moved to an apartment. Our youngest son was having anger issues and was living with his father. I was always concerned about him and felt lost that I couldn't help him. I was stressed beyond belief. Less than a year later my husband and I were divorced.

By 1990 I had an okay job and also ran my own accounting business part time. My finances were good but I was still stressed and was not eating properly. I began having pains in my chest and back. My doctor determined that I needed my gallbladder removed. After the surgery I started feeling better and my life started to feel normal again.

Dating was a disaster. When I stopped searching for "Mr. Right", I realized that my best friend, John, was the love of my life. He had three wonderful children, Melissa, John II, and Elizabeth. In 1995 John and I married and bought a small home in Reno. We became a blended family with five children, who were by then nearly adults and most living on their own. In 1997 we sold our Reno home and purchased 2 ½ acres with a home that needed a lot of tender loving care 50 miles east of Reno. On our land we grew our own vegetables as organically as we were able. Over the years we expanded our farm to 10 acres and had chickens, ducks, milking goats, horses, peacocks, cats and dogs. We loved how we lived and were on our way to becoming self sufficient. We got all our milk from our goats and made cheese and goat milk soap. Our chickens and ducks provided eggs. Our garden was bountiful each year so we canned what we were unable to eat fresh. We canned pickles from our cucumbers, canned or froze our corn, peas, carrots and beans. We canned tomatoes which also yielded a variety of wonderful tomato sauces and juice. We distilled our water and installed a solar water heater.

The biggest drawback to living on a farm was that our jobs were in Reno and we had to commute 100 miles roundtrip every day. My husband was the head of the carpenters training center and I was the controller and secretary/treasurer to the largest roofing company in Northern Nevada. Before the economic crisis in 2008, the company employed over 300 people, had offices in Elko and Carson City, Nevada as well as Portola, California. I was responsible for all accounting department locations, including the home office in Sparks, Nevada. My job was stressful, but I loved it.

Stress is a big part of illness but many people do not recognize it as a potential problem. It may have lead to my many health problems. In 2004 I was hospitalized for possible heart attack, which was eventually diagnosed as angina. In 2006 I had a benign breastbone tumor removed. In 2008 I had a benign neuroma (tumor) removed from my right foot.

And in 2011 I was diagnosed with the big "C"—Triple Negative Breast Cancer of my left breast. Shortly after the cancer diagnosis a tumor on my pituitary was discovered. These were all signs of ill health possibly caused by stress and I failed to recognize them as symptoms.

I didn't know how all these health problems could happen to me, especially cancer. I thought I was eating well. I had no bad habits such as smoking or drinking to excess. We lived on a farm, grew our own vegetables and did it as organically as possible. I made my own bread, occasionally ate potato chips, pizza, French fries, and other fried foods. I gained weight but I still thought I ate well because the bad foods were not in excess. I developed asthma and was put on inhalers; my cholesterol went through the roof and was put on statins; I had acid reflux and was put on Prilosec; and I had bouts of insomnia. My body was telling me that something was terribly wrong and I did not listen. I thought perhaps it was environmental. I don't know specifically about that either, but environmental factors may have contributed due to what I know now. But one thing I do know, my body was unwell. It was making tumors and I had to stop it. It took cancer to make me "wake up" and change!

I was originally devastated by the breast cancer diagnosis and had no idea that there were several types of breast cancer. I thought breast cancer was just breast cancer, period. I was told there is no guarantee of a cancer cure. Not even the "standard" conventional cancer treatments state there is a cure. I was told if I did not do chemotherapy and/or radiation, statistically I would not live past twelve months. There was also no guarantee I wouldn't get cancer again.

What I have gone through and what I have learned, my life without the "standard treatments" has been healthier and my chances of being cancer free, I believe, have multiplied tenfold. For this reason I wrote "An Awakening to Health Cookbook." It is a separate book that contains healthy recipes based on what I learned during my two years of healing and hope to have it released soon in 2016.

Being diagnosed with breast cancer and living past my "statistical" life expectancy of twelve months has made me determined to share my story. I really want to emphasize to everyone the importance of healthy lifestyle changes whether it is cancer, diabetes, pancreatic disease, or any chronic disease for that matter.

Part I

The Discovery, Diagnosis and Treatments

Chapter One

The Discovery

I WAS IN MY LATE FORTIES WHEN I began receiving yearly mammograms. Nothing was ever detected in any of my tests. In 2010 the U.S. Preventive Services Task Force released a final breast cancer screening publication recommending biennial mammography screening for women 50-74 years. Based on that report, I skipped my 2010 test.

In mid-July 2011 I noticed a lump in my left breast while doing my monthly self breast exam. I had never had lumps prior to this and was concerned enough to want to schedule a doctor appointment. But, I also did not want to alarm my husband so I elected not to tell him until after I had gone to the doctor. However, I procrastinated making the call out of fear.

One evening in bed my husband reached over to cuddle me. He was startled to discover the lump and asked if I knew about it. I told him I did and that I planned to call for an appointment. I told him not to worry. He was appalled that I hadn't told him or even obtained an appointment after two weeks of my discovery.

Ironically, the next day, August 1, I got a letter in the mail stating my coverage as a dependent under my husband's health insurance was cancelled effective August 1. The letter went on to say that since I was turning 65 at the end of August I should have already applied for Medicare under Social Security. Holy crap! Now what?!

I flung the letter on the table and immediately called the insurance company. I argued that I was cancelled the same day I received the letter of cancellation and that the letter was dated August 1. I was then told, "You know when your birthday is so you should have known your age for Medicare eligibility." I was not only upset, but humiliated by the insurance coordinators response. He then cited the page where I could read the policy myself. He further told me that I should have applied for Medicare two months ago. I was so outraged I barked back, "I have never reached this age before and I should have received something in the mail BEFORE my coverage was cancelled." Of course my words were to no avail.

The following day I went to the Social Security office in Reno and signed up for Medicare, which was effective immediately. This was good I thought, until I discovered Medicare is like catastrophe insurance. I needed a supplemental policy to cover the deductibles, co-insurance, and charges that could occur in excess of approved Medicare payment amounts. To make things even more frustrating, I needed a separate prescription drug policy—all of which wouldn't be in effect until September 1. Now we were faced with paying monthly insurance premiums for Medicare, supplemental insurance, prescription drug insurance as well as continuing to pay the monthly premiums related to my husband's insurance. What a nightmare.

We made a decision to call the doctor with only the Medicare coverage in place. The next morning I scheduled the earliest available appointment in mid-August. Waiting for this appointment caused anxiety with the "what if" scenarios that were constantly running through my head and I was still quite nervous when the appointment finally arrived. During the appointment the doctor examined my breast and concluded the lump was significant and ordered a mammogram and an ultrasound. She said if the mammogram revealed that an ultrasound was required, an approval from the radiologist would be immediately granted. She then informed me that she would be leaving on a two week vacation but would tell the on-call doctor about my situation. She assured me there was probably nothing to worry about as this was a normal protocol.

The mammogram itself can be a very uncomfortable procedure and sometimes I had pain because my breasts are dense. I expressed my concerns to my doctor. She rummaged through her exam room desk drawers and found a pamphlet with information that I could do to minimize the pain.

What to do to minimize mammogram pain

Limit Caffeine prior to the exam: Caffeine exacerbates the feeling of fullness of dense breasts and triggers cysts to be active. If breasts are tender after consuming caffeine, for example if it is painful to hug, cut out caffeine for up to a week before the mammogram appointment.

Type of breast tissue: Fibro glandular breast tissue is a little more sensitive than fatty tissue. Nothing can be done about the type of tissue you have, but that's something that a mammography technician will take into consideration when she personalizes the mammogram.

Time of cycle: breasts may be more sensitive just before the menstrual cycle so schedule the mammogram appointment after that time of the month.

Fear: Relax! Don't think too much about the procedure itself. If there is a fear of getting a mammogram, being tense will activate an exaggerated feeling from every touch.

Armed with this information, I stopped drinking anything that was caffeinated. I didn't have menstrual cycle any longer so that was not an issue. My mammogram was scheduled on Friday, September 2, 2011 at 9:30 in the morning. That morning I did some relaxing meditation before arriving at my appointment. Upon my arrival I was immediately checked in and was directed to a waiting room different from the main lobby where my husband was asked to wait. I didn't have to wait long before a nurse took me to a changing room and ask me to undress from the waist up and put on a short gown. My socks, shoes, and pants were left on.

A female technician then escorted me to the mammogram room where I was placed to stand in front of a machine. My gown was lowered off my shoulders and my arms were placed in various positions above my head with a bar to hold onto so I wouldn't move. The first image was to be taken with the machine level so my left breast was placed in the center of the bottom imaging plate. Stickers were then placed on the nipple and other places on the breasts so the radiologist could easily identify the nipples and any moles in the final images. An imaging arm came down that covered the entire breast that squeezed my breast flat as possible so an image could be taken. Once the image was taken the arm was raised and the pressure was released. A second image was taken with the machine tilted for a different angle using the same technique to obtain an image. I found this mammogram experience to be more uncomfortable than painful this time. I attributed this to be better because I did not drink any caffeine the entire week before the mammogram and did meditation that morning.

On my previous mammograms I was asked to get dressed go home and wait for the results from my doctor or by mail in a couple of weeks. However, this time I was asked to wait in a different room with my husband until the radiologist reviewed the images. Before she left the room she told me that the radiologist may want more images taken because my breasts were dense and dense breasts are harder to read so more images must be taken and not to be alarmed. After she left the room my husband and I looked at each other, took a deep breath, sat, and waited. A few minutes later the radiologist entered and said she ordered an ultrasound immediately as the lump looked suspicious. "Oh crap!" I thought. Now I was really afraid.

I asked many questions about the ultrasound. The technician told me it was a noninvasive medical test that helps physicians diagnose and treat medical conditions. It was safe and painless and ultrasound uses sound waves to produce pictures of the inside of the body and there is no radiation exposure to the patient. The ultrasound images are captured in real-time and can show the structure and movement of the body's internal organs as well as blood flowing through blood vessels.

With that, I was escorted to the ultrasound room where I undressed from the waist up. I was asked to lie on my back on the examining table and raise my left arm above my head. After I was positioned on the exam table, the radiologist applied a warm water-based gel (the gel does not stain or discolor clothing) to the area of the breast being studied. The technician explained that the gel helps the transducer (wand-like instrument) make a secure contact with the breast and it eliminates air pockets between the transducer and the skin that can block the sound waves from passing into the body. She placed the transducer on my breast and moved it back and forth over my breast until the desired images were captured. I experienced no discomfort from pressure as the transducer was pressed against my breast. Once the imaging was complete, she wiped the clear ultrasound gel off my skin.

After the ultrasound, my husband and I were escorted to a private room to wait for the results. Waiting was unbearable and hours seemed to pass. In reality it was only twenty minutes before the radiologist and her assistant came back to our room. The radiologist said the ultrasound results appeared to be suspicious and suggested it would be prudent to obtain an approval from my doctor for an immediate biopsy. Again, the word "suspicious". What is it with this word? I advised her that my doctor was on vacation for another week and no approval could be obtained until then. The radiologist took my hand, stepped in front of me, looked directly into my eyes and insisted I needed to have a biopsy done immediately.

I felt an overwhelming feeling of fear and began to shake. I felt my eyes fill and tears roll down my checks. She spoke quietly, tried to calm me, and gently requested her assistant to get a nurse navigator assigned to me immediately to be my advocate. She explained that a nurse navigator is a person who assists in the process of getting emergency approval and acts on a patient's behalf. A navigator would help with any questions and concerns I might have. The radiologist instructed us to go to lunch. If approval was granted, she would call me on my cell phone. Within two hours the proper approvals were obtained and we were asked to come back as a biopsy was scheduled that very afternoon.

I felt sick to my stomach. Just the thought of having the biopsy was very scary. Upon my return I was immediately escorted to the same changing room and ask to undress from the waist up and put on a short gown. My socks, shoes, and pants were again left on.

For the biopsy I was brought to an exam room much like the ultrasound room. I was instructed to lie on my back on the exam table and position my arms at my side. My left breast was wiped with a sanitizing swab and I was injected with a substance to numb the area of the breast to be biopsied.

There are many types of breast biopsy procedures. I received a **core needle biopsy.** This type of breast biopsy is used to assess a breast lump that's visible on a mammogram or ultrasound or that the doctor feels during a clinical breast exam.

Once the breast area was numbed, the radiologist used a thin hollow needle to remove a tissue sample using ultrasound guidance. Several samples were collected to be analyzed. I was bandaged, instructed to get dressed, and then escorted back to the waiting room.

By this point I was a nervous wreck. A nurse came in later and said that since it was Labor Day weekend the results might not be available until the following Tuesday depending on what was discovered. With that information we went home.

Since nothing else could be done except to wait, my husband decided to pack our camper and truck and take me on a camping trip over the long three-day holiday. He wanted us to focus on more positive and happy thoughts. We forgot about the biopsy and had a wonderful time camping and hiking. We returned late Monday and since I had not received a call regarding the biopsy results, I was feeling optimistic.

Chapter Two

The Diagnosis

TUESDAY MORNING I DECIDED TO GO to work. I was dressed and ready to leave when I received a phone call. The caller identified herself as a hospital scheduler and wanted to schedule an emergency surgery. I asked her, "Why do I need surgery?" I didn't understand the call. There was a long pause before she asked, "Have you been contacted by your doctor?" I said I hadn't and asked again, "Why do I need surgery?" She requested that I contact my doctor about the results of the biopsy. I felt a sinking feeling in the pit of my stomach and asked, "Is this for cancer?" Again there was no reply. I asked again, "Are you saying I have cancer?" She then replied, "You have to speak to your doctor." I felt weak. My knees started to buckle and I felt I was going to vomit. My husband heard the alarm in my voice. He immediately came into the room and wanted to know what was going on. The look on his face was as scary to me as the voice on the phone. His eyes were wide with fear. I hung up the phone, sat down, and said, "I think I have cancer." We both just sat there and stared at each other not saying a word and I started to cry.

After I composed myself, I called my doctor and was told she had not yet returned from her vacation. I explained to the receptionist what happened and left word to have the on-call doctor or my doctor to call me immediately.

Hours had passed and it was early afternoon and still there was no word. Our daughter called to find out about the biopsy. I told her what had happened and she reminded us that I was assigned a nurse navigator and to call her. The navigator was wonderful. She said she'd find out what was going on and set up an appointment to meet with her at 4:30 that very afternoon.

When we arrived, she had a huge three-ring binder filled with all kinds of information. As we paged through the book she explained that I had been diagnosed with triple negative breast cancer of the left breast and what would happen next. The book was full of questions to ask doctors and places to write the answers. It had blank appointment pages and spaces for diagnoses and reports as well as card holders for doctors' business cards. She explained the book would be almost like my "bible." It included steps that I would be going through, doctors I would be seeing, procedures, and surgery information. It was amazing! But I couldn't help but feel angry. I was angry the way I found out about my cancer diagnosis.

Triple negative breast cancer

The next day I started to research triple negative breast cancer (TNBC) and prepared myself for the worst. It is a very invasive, fast-growing ductile cancer that is difficult to treat. It is the deadliest breast cancer. It doesn't have biomarkers (a biomarker refers to measurable indicators) for the estrogen receptor (ER), progesterone receptor (PR), or the human epidermal growth factor receptor 2 (HER2) proteins, hence the term "triple-negative." Without these biomarkers, TNBC is more difficult to treat since most chemotherapies target one of the three receptors and TNBC has poorer prognosis than hormone receptor positive breast cancers.

Breast cancer is the most common cancer in women worldwide. In 2011 it was estimated that over one million new cases would be diagnosed. From that, approximately 15% would be classified as triple-negative. TNBC is mostly found among women who carry a mutation in the BRCA1 gene (breast cancer susceptibility gene 1) or BRCA2 gene (breast cancer susceptibility gene 2). Up to 20% of patients with TNBC have a BRCA mutation, particularly in the BRCA1 gene. I was tested for both these genes and do not have it.

TNBC is more commonly diagnosed in younger African American women, who are less than 45 years of age. Out of the 15% of women diagnosed with TNBC, only 10% are white. It is most uncommon that a white woman of my age, 65, be diagnosed with this type of cancer.

Since the three protein biomarkers for, ER, PR and HER2, represent the only known targets for breast cancer treatment currently, a considerable amount of effort has been made to better understand the driving forces of TNBC. Unfortunately at this time, there has been discouraging preliminary clinical data regarding TNBC. The "standard" chemotherapy remains the most common form of treatment for TNBC. And, because TNBC tends to be more aggressive, it gets a more aggressive treatment. But, it is important for cancer patients to understand how doctors use a pathology report to determine what treatment to use for different breast cancers.

What is a pathology report?

A pathology report is a written medical record of a tissue diagnosis. A pathology report for breast cancer includes the results of a hormone receptor assay. This test tells whether or not the breast cancer cells have receptors for the hormones estrogen and progesterone. Hormone receptors are proteins that are found in and on breast cells that pick up hormone signals telling the cells to grow. If it has receptors for estrogen, this type of cancer is called **estrogen-receptor-positive** (or ER). In this case the cancer cells, like normal breast cells, may receive signals from estrogen that could promote their growth. If a cancer is **progesterone-receptor-positive** (PR) it has progesterone receptors. Again, this means that the cancer cells may receive signals from progesterone that could promote their growth. The same is true for human epidermal growth factor receptor 2 (HER2) proteins. Roughly two out of every three breast cancers test positive for hormone receptors. Testing for hormone receptors is important because the results help the doctor decide whether the cancer is likely to respond to hormonal therapy or other treatments. Estrogen promotes the growth of cancers that are hormone receptor-positive. Hormonal therapy includes medications that either lower the amount of estrogen in the body or block estrogen from supporting the growth and function of breast cells. If the breast cancer cells have hormone receptors, then hormone-based chemotherapy could help slow or stop their growth.

This is what the inside of a breast looks like

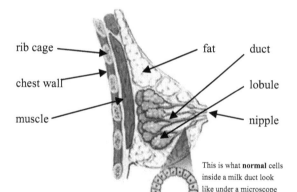

rib cage — fat   duct

chest wall   lobule

muscle   nipple

This is what **normal** cells inside a milk duct look like under a microscope

Image retrieved from http://www.breastcancer.org/pictures/breast_anatomy/axillary_lymph_nodes

If the cancer is **hormone-receptor-negative** (no receptors are present), then hormonal therapy will not work. I do not have any receptors so none of the hormonal therapy would work for me.

Now that I understood my type of cancer diagnosis, it was time for me to meet the surgeon since surgery is usually the first line of attack against breast cancer.

I met with the surgeon that was recommended by my primary physician. We discussed my medical history and he barraged me with a series of questions. My surgeon was very thorough and asked that I not hold back any information, even if I thought it was irrelevant or embarrassing. He said the answers were extremely important and were to be answered truthfully as possible because some medications can have serious effects on my body's ability to handle the shock of surgery and heal well afterwards. I explained all my past bad reactions to procedures, medications, and allergies. We discussed drugs I was currently taking that were prescribed, non-prescribed, as well as vitamins and herbal supplements I was taking. I was asked to stop taking aspirin and any non-steroidal anti-inflammatory medications, such as ibuprofen, garlic and onions several weeks before surgery as these can promote excessive bleeding during surgery. We discussed what the surgery involves, the preparation, risks, and recovery. We discussed that if good clean margins were unattainable (no cancer cells seen at the outer edge of the tissue that was removed) that a total mastectomy would be probable followed by chemotherapy and radiation. We discussed further the severity of this type of breast cancer and he recommended I see an oncologist after my recovery. On September 21, 2011, I was scheduled to have a partial mastectomy, also called a lumpectomy.

Chapter Three

The Surgery and Unconventional Therapy

I HAD TO CHECK IN FOUR HOURS EARLY at the hospital the day of my surgery, to undergo special procedures to prepare for surgery. After I checked in and completed the necessary paperwork, I was brought to a changing room and asked to put on a hospital gown and booties. My clothes, shoes and other personal belongings were placed in a plastic bag. A sticker with my name and hospital information for identification purposes was affixed to the bag. A nurse then escorted me to a small room with a gurney-like bed where my husband was nervously waiting in a chair next to the bed. My bag of personal items was placed on a rack under the bed. The nurse took my blood pressure, temperature and pulse, noted the information and said a technician would be coming to get me for an MRI. She said that because I have dense breasts an MRI was ordered and the results of the images would help my surgeon plan the best approach for my surgery and my treatment plan after surgery. The technician came in shortly after my vitals were taken and brought me into a room with a huge machine. I was instructed to lie on my stomach with my breasts aligned through holes on the bed of the machine. A set of sound proof head phones was put over my ears and I was slid into the machine so images could then be taken of my breasts. Even though I had headphones on, the machine was still very loud.

After this procedure I had another special procedure, a sentinel node biopsy. This was to find the sentinel lymph node. The sentinel lymph node is the very first lymph node in which cancer cells are most likely to spread from the primary tumor. This node is an important node to locate as it determines if cancer has spread beyond the primary tumor into the lymphatic system. I found this procedure to be very difficult, emotionally stressful, embarrassing and humiliating. My gown was lowered to my waist and I was placed in a reclining chair. A male technician cleansed my left breast with a sanitizing solution then injected a numbing substance above my nipple and then directly into my nipple, which was most painful. Then a tracer material made up of radioactive isotope was injected directly into my nipple. The radioactive isotope follows up the armpit through the blood stream and during surgery a device is used to detect radioactivity to find the sentinel node to be removed. The node is then checked for the presence of cancer cells by a pathologist. My sentinel node and three other nodes were removed which were in axillary lymph nodes as shown in level II.

Lymph Node Areas Adjacent to Breast Area

    A Pectoralis major muscle
    B Axillary lymph nodes: level
    C Axillary lymph nodes: level II
    D Axillary lymph nodes: level III
    E Supraclavicular lymph nodes
    F Internal mammary lymph nodes

Image retrieved from http://www.breastcancer.org/pictures/breast_anatomy/axillary_lymph_nodes

Another procedure was done at the same time as the sentinel node biopsy, called a wire-localization or needle-localization. A radiologist used an ultrasound to guide and insert a very thin wire into the breast in the area of the cancer. The surgeon would use this wire as a guide to find and remove the tumor during surgery. When this last procedure was completed I was brought back to the small gurney bedroom where my husband was still waiting. A nurse came in and began to administer an IV (intravenous) for anesthesia and other drugs that would be given to me during surgery. The anesthesiologist then came in, introduced himself and asked me questions about my allergies and drug reactions and tried to make me feel relaxed about the procedure. The more he tried to relax me the more I became nervous. Finally my surgeon came in and said everything was ready and he'd do his best to save as much of my breast as he could but also said that there was a chance I'd have to have a full mastectomy. I told him that I knew and was ready to get it over with. He shook my husband's hand and said he'd speak with him after surgery. My husband bent down to hug, kiss me, and finally he squeezed my hand before he left to the waiting room.

During surgery I was administered general anesthesia, which means I was asleep during the surgery. An incision was made in the breast to remove the tumor along with normal tissue surrounding the tumor. Because of the location and the size of the tumor much more of the breast tissue had to be removed in order to get good, clean, margins. A margin is described as negative or clean when the pathologist finds no cancer cells at the edge of the tissue, suggesting that all the cancer has been removed. My surgeon was able to get good margins to within 3mm of my breast bone. The incision was then closed with stitches. The surgery made my left breast smaller than the right and the nipple had to be relocated which was higher than my right breast. My surgeon also made an incision in the underarm area and removed the four lymph nodes to be tested for cancer. Luckily they were clear of cancer. Drain tubes were inserted to drain body fluid such as pus, blood or other fluids from the incision which could accumulate and cause infection. I was hospitalized overnight and sent home the next day with the drains which would be removed at my post-op visit two weeks after surgery.

Two weeks after I had my post-op surgery visit, I met with an oncologist. He instructed me on the steps I needed to take following my surgery recovery which included chemotherapy and radiation. According to him chemotherapy and radiation were the only way to treat this type of cancer. I requested to wait before committing to this treatment so I could research and learn more about the types of treatment. He wasn't happy about my decision to wait but agreed. His parting words were, "You can wait only a few more weeks to "knock" this out. This is a very aggressive cancer."

I took a few weeks to research my options while I healed from surgery. The first couple of weeks in October I visited an integrative medical center that combines allopathic (conventional medicine) and holistic medicine specializing in cancer. The center's approach involved administering a very low dose of insulin targeted IV chemotherapy with vitamins. The goal of low-dose or metronomic dosing is not given in cycles like the standard chemotherapy. Instead, it is given in smaller amounts daily, for a longer period of time. Metronomic dosing does not destroy tumor cells but it kills the endothelial cells—the cells that line the inside of the blood and lymph vessels. These endothelial cells create the blood vessels that tumors need to flourish, grow, and to metastasize to other locations. By killing the endothelial cells, metronomic dosing aims to stop angiogenesis (angio means "vessels," and genesis means "growth") or sometimes referred to as anti-angiogenic chemotherapy. These cells are attractive target cells because they do not mutate and become cancer-resistant in the way that tumor cells do. However, I rejected the chemotherapy until I could understand more about this type of treatment and its side effects but agreed to two weeks of intravenous vitamins to boost my immune system which would be considered unconventional therapy.

My main immune boosting protocol included vitamin C, B vitamins and glutathione. I was administered high dose vitamin C via an IV. High dose vitamin C has an anti-viral, anti-bacterial, and anti-cancer effect. It is very helpful in preventing growing tumors from invading other tissue and boosts the activation of natural killer (NK) cells so that the immune system has extra armor to protect against diseases, including cancer. NK cells are a type of white blood cells that are critical to the innate immune system and are among the many essential components involved in fighting cancer. However, vitamin C must be administered in large amounts. Hence the term, "High Dose". High doses of vitamin C also boost the body's ability to produce interferon, another anti-cancer agent.

I also received vitamins B6, B complex—B1, B2, B3, B5, B6, B7, B9—and B12 through the IV port. These vitamins play a key role in synthesizing antibodies that are needed to fight various diseases. They can reduce inflammation and are important for healthy functioning of muscles, nerves, and heart while regulating the nervous and digestive systems, helping normal cell growth and development, and producing hormones. These vitamins support the immune system and aid the body in breaking down protein. B9, helps cells make and maintain DNA, which may help prevent breast cancer, colorectal cancer, and pancreatic cancer. B12 may lower cervical cancer risk and reduce levels of homocysteine (an amino acid thought to contribute to heart disease when it occurs at elevated levels).

Vitamin B-17 (Laetrile) was also put through the IV port. It is not harmful on normal cells but is deadly to cancer cells because Laetrile works by targeting and killing cancer cells and building the immune system to fend off future outbreaks of cancer.

I also received Glutathione through the IV port. It is a protein that is found inside every cell of the human body, with the highest concentrations found in the liver. It acts as a powerful antioxidant and detoxifier that protects cells from free radicals and oxidative stress and boosts the immune system.

During my time receiving immune boosting IV vitamins, I met some amazing people receiving cancer treatments. One woman that really made me emotional was from the Seattle area and was diagnosed with an inoperable brain cancer. Her condition had gone undiagnosed for six months by the medical profession. Her husband described her condition as being so degenerated that she was nearly comatose. Her situation was so bad that doctors told the family there was no hope and nothing further could be done; she was sent home to die. In desperation her family members searched until they discovered a facility that offered an alternative treatment approach. When they arrived a week earlier, his wife was wheeled in to the integrative facility on a gurney, barely conscious.

When I first met her she was sitting up in a reclining chair and conversing with her husband and adult daughter. Her family had to speak slowly with her, although her responses were remedial, she *was* communicating. They were thrilled that there was such great improvement in such a short period of time. The unconventional therapy she received was the IV treatments of high dose vitamin C, trace minerals and other components (which were not told to me). The treatments were considered non-toxic, and integrated with conventional medicines that somehow targeted the disease while boosting her immune system. The husband was truly grateful of his wife's progress. I can attest to the fact that each time my husband and I saw her she was considerably better. The final time I saw her she acknowledged me for the first time with a head nod and a smile when her husband spoke. I couldn't look directly at her after that as I felt a tear roll down my cheek.

During my treatments at the center I also met a young man in his early twenties. He was being treated for brain cancer. He and his parents had come from Germany seeking an alternative treatment approach as the conventional treatment given him was not working. Speaking in broken English, his parents conveyed that their son had already gone through two weeks of his three week intensive "Cancer Boot Camp" therapy at the center. They felt it was a miracle to have such a wonderful thing that could extend their son's life. He had already made such headway compared to what he had been going through before coming to the center. I saw him only twice before he left for home and each time I could see how much better he was doing just talking and walking.

These two people touched me so emotionally because I began to realize that I too had hope for a cure.

When I completed the immune boosting treatments, I returned to my oncologist and requested a second opinion. He agreed and set up an appointment with another oncologist on November 2, 2011, at the University of California, Davis. I wanted to find out about the available treatment programs at UC Davis and what they could do for me.

Chapter Four

Oncologists

THE UC DAVIS CANCER HOSPITAL was a three hour drive so we stayed overnight with our son in San Ramon, California. The next morning we arrived at the hospital. I was very apprehensive and afraid about the appointment as I did not know what to expect. I tried to remain positive but the visit at UC Davis was not received well by me. I felt I was a number and not a person. My husband and I stood for 45 minutes in a huge line just to sign in for my appointment. I tried to turn in my written diagnoses and some tumor slides from my surgery that I brought to be reviewed. I was told they already had the information and to show the doctor that was scheduled to see me.

We waited with my packet in hand for another hour before being escorted to an exam room. Then we waited another thirty minutes before I was actually seen. When the oncologist finally made it to the exam room, her first words were not hello or even to introduce herself, but, "Why are you here?" I told her about my cancer diagnosis and desire to get another treatment recommendation. "So I am the second opinion doctor then." she said. When I confirmed her statement she finally introduced herself, stated her position and credentials. As she shook hands with us I handed her my packet of information and tumor slides. She sat, placed them on her lap, and proceeded to explain the standard protocol at UC Davis. She recommended a chemotherapy treatment followed by radiation due to the seriousness of my type of cancer. She emphasized that without any kind of "standard" treatment I could perhaps live six to twelve months.

I did not feel comfortable with her recommendation. I was hoping for a different solution as this was the same information I was told by my first oncologist. I let her know I wanted to do more research about the treatment. She became indignant and handed my packet and slides back without reviewing the contents. We were then excused. The entire appointment was about fifteen or twenty minutes and I wasn't even examined! I felt the entire trip was a waste of time. By the time we left the building, I was totally devastated and never wanted to return. I didn't understand the doctor's attitude. I felt afraid, alone, and in total despair. I thought I was surely going to die. I cried most of the three hour drive home and became very depressed.

I went back to work the next week and tried to do the best I could to maintain my composure throughout my usual workdays. I tried to prepare myself for the worst. I started to cut my hair a couple of inches at a time. Soon my waist-length hair reached my mid-back and I was even ready to make an appointment to have it shaved and made into a wig. I was desperate for help and felt I had no other choice but to do whatever I was told by the doctors.

My husband's brother, an MD, was concerned with my diagnoses and came to visit. He and his wife, a nurse, gave us advice and tried to help with my decision. I said I wanted to find out more and that I was still very afraid of chemotherapy. He was sympathetic and used his professional contacts to connect me with an oncologist at the Stanford Cancer Center in Palo Alto, California.

On December 29, 2011, after a five hour drive, my husband and I met with the Assistant Professor of Oncology Medicine at the Stanford University Medical Center. She was the administrator of the Scientific

Program Committee for Triple Negative Breast Cancer Therapy of the American Society of Clinical Oncology. H-o-l-y cow! My brother-in-law got me an appointment with the best!

I spent a long exhausting day at the cancer center. We arrived at ten in the morning. I was examined for about an hour with one doctor before I actually met the TNBC oncologist. She was amazing and I was in her care another two hours during examinations, blood tests and consultations about chemotherapy treatments. Because the oncologist listened to all of my concerns and worries that I would die from the chemotherapy rather than cancer, she recommended that I attend a nutrition consultation. She further stated that nutrition and exercise were two areas in which lifestyle changes could help reduce the risk of recurrent or new cancers and promote survival.

We spent the night again with our son and discussed the appointment. The next morning we went home and waited until an appointment could be arranged with a nutritional counselor. When an appointment was finally arranged, my husband and I returned to Stanford and attended the nutrition counseling together. There we learned the value of the Mediterranean diet and how important a lifestyle change is—especially for a cancer diagnosis.

After the nutritional counseling, I saw the Stanford oncologist again later that same day to discuss my treatment options. She still recommended that I undergo some type of "standard" cancer chemotherapy. However, she felt it would be best combined with diet lifestyle changes to help the immune system during chemotherapy treatments. We discussed how systemic chemotherapy could reduce the risk of recurrence and how the adjuvant method could increase the likelihood of long-term survival. Adjuvant therapy uses an additional drug, usually given after surgery where all detectable disease has been removed but where there remains a "statistical" risk of relapse of the disease. Basically one drug is added to enhance the other as a combination therapy. Adjuvant therapy was estimated to have 12% absolute benefit in terms of my mortality and 18% benefit in terms of cancer relapse. I was uncomfortable with these percentage odds. I would have preferred the percentages to have been at least 50% in terms of mortality and relapse. The fear of chemotherapy was still strong within me. Understanding my reluctance of taking drugs due to my severe reactions to multiple different medications, the Stanford oncologist recommended five chemotherapy options. They ranged from the most aggressive chemotherapy, which she preferred and insisted upon, to the minimum chemotherapy or radiation requirements which she felt was better than nothing.

All three oncologists I saw stressed that the most aggressive form of therapy would be the most beneficial and would kill any rogue cancer cells left in my body. They cited studies that have shown that TNBC is more likely to spread beyond the breast and more likely to recur after treatment and that the five-year survival rates also tend to be lower for TNBC patients. This information didn't make me feel comfortable at all about doing chemotherapy.

We discussed that TNBC recurrence happened early in the first one to three years after diagnosis and that *my* survival rate was twelve months without chemotherapy. I learned that the surgery specimen removed was 7cm x 1.8cm and in just 20 days the tumor that was inside the removed specimen had grown from 2.8cm to 3.4cm x 1.8cm and was classified as grade III, Nottingham score 9, which is an aggressive dividing cell, and with zero cancer found in the four axillary lymph nodes that were removed, the cancer was evaluated as stage II, invasive ductal carcinoma, triple negative breast cancer. I was told the risks and how important it was that I do some kind of chemotherapy as soon as possible. But, what are grades, scores and stages?

Grades

Grade is a "score" that tells how different the appearance and growth patterns of cancer cells are from those of normal, healthy breast cells. The cancer is rated on a scale from 1 to 3. In Grade I or low grade (sometimes also called well differentiated), the cancer cells look a little bit different from normal cells, and they grow in slow, well-organized patterns. Not many cells are dividing to make new cancer cells. In Grade

II or intermediate/moderate grade (moderately differentiated), the cancer cells do not look like normal cells and are growing and dividing a little faster than normal. Cell growth and division is difficult to explain. When the normal balance between cell division and cell loss is disrupted the basal cells divide faster than needed to replenish the cells being shed, and with each division both of the two newly formed cells will often retain the capacity to divide, leading to an increased number of dividing cells. This creates a growing mass of tissue called a "tumor". As more and more dividing cells accumulate, the normal organization of the tissue gradually becomes disrupted. In Grade III or high grade (poorly differentiated), the cancer cells look very different from normal cells. They grow quickly in disorganized, irregular patterns, with many dividing to make new cancer cells. The cancer tumor removed from me was at Grade III.

Scores

Nottingham histological score is simply a scoring system to assess the "grade" of breast cancers. It is a total score based on three different sub-scores. The three sub-scores are assigned based on three components of how the breast cancer cells look under a microscope. (The details of these three components are not critical for understanding.) Each of the three components is assigned sub-scores of 1, 2, or 3; 1 being best and 3 being worst. Once the three sub-scores are added, a Nottingham score is obtained: the minimum score possible is 3 (1+1+1) and the maximum possible is 9 (3+3+3). All three sub-scores on my cancer tumor removed were scored as 3 so it was graded the highest score of 9.

Nottingham scores of 3, 4, and 5 refer to Grade I, scores of 6 and 7 refer to Grade II, and scores of 8 or 9 refer to Grade III. High-score cancers tend to relapse more often than low-score cancers.

Stages of breast cancer

When I attended the Stanford Cancer Clinic, I was given information that explained the stages of breast cancer. The National Cancer Institute's booklet *What You Need to Know about Breast Cancer* describes a stage usually expressed as a number on a scale of 0 through

IV with Stage 0 describing noninvasive cancers that remain within their original location and Stage IV describing invasive cancers that have spread outside the breast to other parts of the body.

Stage 0 Zero is sometimes used to describe abnormal cells that are not invasive cancer. Zero is also used for ductal carcinoma in situ (DCIS). DCIS is diagnosed when abnormal cells have not invaded nearby breast tissue or spread outside the duct. Doctors at times don't consider DCIS to be cancer which sometimes becomes invasive breast cancer if not treated.

Stage I describes the breast cancer as cancer cells that have invaded normal surrounding breast tissue, the tumor measures up to two centimeters, and the cancer has not spread outside the breast. Microscopic invasion is possible in stage I breast cancer. In microscopic invasion, the cancer cells have just started to invade the tissue outside the lining of the duct or lobule, but the invading cancer cells do not measure more than one millimeter.

Stage II describes invasive breast cancer in which the tumor is not more than two centimeters and cancer has spread to the lymph nodes under the arm or, the tumor is between two and five centimeters and the cancer has not spread to the lymph nodes under the arm or, the tumor is between two and five centimeters and the cancer has spread to the lymph nodes under the arm or, the tumor is larger than five centimeters and the cancer has not spread to the lymph nodes under the arm.

Stage III is locally advanced cancer and is divided into subcategories known as IIIA, IIIB, and IIIC.

Stage IIIA describes invasive breast cancer in which either the tumor is no more than five centimeters and cancer has spread to underarm lymph nodes that are attached to each other or to other structures or, the cancer may have spread to lymph nodes behind the breastbone and the tumor is more than five centimeters and the cancer has spread to the underarm lymph nodes that are either alone or attached to each other or to other structures or, the cancer may have spread to lymph nodes behind the breastbone.

Stage IIIB describes invasive breast cancer tumor of any size that has grown into the chest wall or the skin of the breast. It may be associated with swelling of the breast or with lumps in the breast skin, the cancer may have spread to lymph nodes under the arm, the cancer may have spread to the underarm lymph nodes that are attached to each other or other structures or, the cancer may have spread to lymph nodes behind the breastbone. Inflammatory breast cancer is considered rare. Typical features of inflammatory breast cancer include reddening of a large portion of the breast skin and the breast feels warm and may be swollen and cancer cells have spread to the lymph nodes and may be found in the skin.

Stage IIIC describes invasive breast cancer tumor of any size and the cancer has spread to lymph nodes above or below the collarbone or, the cancer has spread to axillary lymph nodes or, the cancer has spread to lymph nodes behind the breastbone.

Stage IV describes invasive breast cancer that has spread beyond the breast and the cancer has spread to nearby lymph nodes to other organs of the body, such as the lungs, distant lymph nodes, skin, bones, liver, or brain which are usually terminal. Stage IV uses words such as "advanced" and "metastatic". Cancer may be Stage IV at first diagnosis or it can be a recurrence of a previous breast cancer that has spread to other parts of the body.

I felt pressured by doctors to have chemotherapy treatments. I argued with each of them that in my view, the tumor had been removed through a partial mastectomy with good margins and no cancer was present in the removed lymph nodes and I was diagnosed stage II and not yet in the stage III. However, because my tumor was a grade III and a Nottingham score 9, the oncologists feared that the cancer would come back after a partial mastectomy (lumpectomy). This is the highest grade and there is significant history of recurrence in post lumpectomy. Therefore based on my age and other factors, the oncologists recommended that I have whole breast radiation after chemotherapy and if a recurrence happened after treatment then I should probably have a mastectomy.

Despite my resistance to chemotherapy and radiation, I felt ready to succumb to them. But I still needed to heal from surgery. I felt that doctors could aid my body by removing the tumor and injecting me with chemicals but it didn't necessarily mean my body would heal. I needed to heal my mental outlook and focus on being as positive as possible. I had to heal from within first.

However, during my healing process, while trying to understand chemotherapy, its alleged benefits versus side effects, I became ill. On January 5, 2012 I developed a severe eye infection and had to go to a local hospital emergency room. Because of the severity of the infection I was given a CT scan which at the time appeared to be normal. I was given antibiotics to fight the infection and told to see my primary physician.

A week later I received a follow-up call from the hospital. The nurse inquired as to how I was doing. I told her the infection was gone and I was feeling fine. She was glad to hear that. There was a pause for a brief moment before she continued. There was another reason for the call. She informed me that the CT scan was reviewed again and it revealed a growth. Immediately I became afraid. There was another brief pause before she suggested that I see my primary physician. She said the growth appeared to be unrelated to the infection.

Now I was stressed again and all kinds of things popped into my mind. What else did I need to go through? Would this be cancer too? Should I do chemotherapy? Should I do radiation? Should I have a complete mastectomy? The caller said it may be nothing serious but said it was important enough for me to contact my primary physician. I thanked her for the call and immediately called my doctor and got an appointment in mid-January, 2012.

My primary physician reviewed the scan and said that I should see a neurologist as there appeared to be a tumor on or near the pituitary gland. She said these tumors are usually benign and not usually a problem. She told me not worry. My immediate thought was, well she said that before and I was diagnosed with cancer. Of course I was apprehensive. She ordered blood tests and referred me to a neurologist.

Chapter Five

Another Diagnosis

IN THE FIRST WEEK OF FEBRUARY, 2012 I met with a neurologist and it was an intense appointment. My husband went with me. After my blood pressure, pulse and temperature was taken he chatted with us awhile and we were able to interview each other. I explained my medical history, surgeries, allergies and my recent cancer diagnosis. I told him I was nervous because we are dealing with my brain and needed to feel comfortable. He smiled and agreed. He told us his credentials, when he became a doctor, why he chose neurology and what his experience was. Then he reviewed my blood test results with us that were ordered by my primary physician. He said the blood tests appeared to be normal. Then we reviewed the scan I had at the hospital and confirmed I had a pituitary tumor. We discussed the probability of various symptoms the tumor may cause and problems associated with pituitary tumors. Pituitary tumors fall into three general categories. The first category is hypersecretion which means too much of any hormone in the body is caused by a secretory (promoting secretion) pituitary tumor. Second, hyposecretion refers to too little of any hormone in the body. This symptom can be caused by a large pituitary tumor, which interferes with the pituitary gland's ability to produce hormones. Hyposecretion can also result from surgery or radiation of the pituitary tumor. A third category refers to tumor mass effects. As a pituitary tumor grows and presses against the pituitary gland or other areas in the brain, it may cause head-aches, vision problems, or other health effects such as dizziness or loss of consciousness.

My recent cancer diagnosis was a concern so he discussed brain surgery with us. He also affirmed that vision problems occur when the tumor "pinches" the nerves that run between the eyes and the brain. Sudden loss of vision, loss of consciousness, and even death can result from sudden bleeding from the tumor.

The idea of brain surgery made me nervous, apprehensive and down-right afraid. I explained I wanted to do research before I committed to brain surgery. He understood and was glad I wanted to find out more. However before my next appointment with him, he wanted me to see a neuroendocrinologist to evaluate the interactions between my hormones and my brain. He also wanted me to see a neuro-ophthalmologist to examine my optic nerve for problems such as inflammation of a peripheral nerve and to evaluate if there was a loss of central vision, side vision or both due to a decreased or interrupted blood flow to the eye's optic nerve. I agreed and appointments were made. I went home to find out more about this type of tumor.

My research indicated that *most* pituitary tumors are noncancerous (benign). Up to 20% of people have pituitary tumors. However, many of these tumors do not cause symptoms and are never diagnosed during a person's lifetime.

The pituitary gland is a tiny organ, the size of a pea, found at the base of the brain. As the master gland or the control panel of the body, it produces many hormones that travel throughout the body, directing certain processes or causing other glands to produce other hormones. The pituitary gland makes or stores many different hormones.

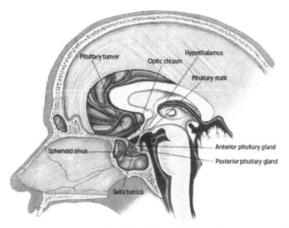

Image retrieved from UCLA Health http://pituitary.ucla.edu/body.cfm?id=47

Pituitary hormones are released in pulses, levels fluctuate during the day, and the release of one hormone directly affects the release of others. Each hormone is released through the bloodstream and affects different organs in the body.

The following hormones and their functions are made in the anterior (front part) of the pituitary gland:

Prolactin - Prolactin stimulates breast milk production after childbirth. It also affects sex hormone levels in women's ovaries and men's testicles. A tumor could be a leading problem to diminished sexual interest, impotence in men as well as fertility.

Growth hormone (GH) - The GH stimulates growth in childhood and is important for maintaining a healthy body composition and well-being in adults. In adults, GH is important for maintaining muscle mass and bone mass. It also affects fat distribution in the body. Acromegaly is a condition that is nearly always caused by a tumor of the pituitary gland. The term acromegaly literally means enlarged extremities.

Adrenocorticotropin (ACTH) - ACTH stimulates the production of cortisol by the adrenal glands—small glands that sit on top of the kidneys. Cortisol, a "stress hormone," is vital to our survival. It helps maintain blood pressure and blood sugar levels, and it is produced in

31

larger amounts when we're under stress, especially after illness or injury. A pituitary tumor can cause changes in ACTH hormonal function. Symptoms include unexpected weight gain, easy bruising of the skin and muscle weakness.

Thyroid-stimulating hormone (TSH) - TSH stimulates the thyroid gland to produce thyroid hormones, which regulate the body's metabolism, energy balance, growth, and nervous system activity. A pituitary tumor that secretes TSH can cause an excess of amount of thyroid hormone that causes hyperthyroidism which can be a serious medical condition.

Luteinizing hormone (LH) - LH stimulates testosterone production in men and ovulation in women.

Follicle-stimulating hormone (FSH) - FSH promotes sperm production in men and stimulates the ovaries to produce estrogen and develop eggs in women. LH and FSH work together to enable normal function of the ovaries and testicles.

I met with the neuroendocrinologist and the neuro-ophthalmologist and had the second appointment with the neurologist. He again discussed surgery to remove the tumor but said all tests revealed no significant problems with my eyesight. However, my hormones needed more testing. I requested a "wait and see approach" and elected not to have surgery right away. The neurologist said before he would agree to wait, he wanted more testing to be done by the neuroendocrinologist.

In mid-March, 2012 I underwent a variety of tests to measure my pituitary hormone levels. My first test would be a dexamethasone suppression test which assesses the function of the adrenal glands. The adrenal glands produce many of the body's hormones and help regulate vital processes. I was prescribed dexamethasone, a pill to take at 11 PM at home the night before the test. I was to take it by mouth, with milk and an antacid to prevent gastric irritation. The dexamethasone measures whether hormone ACTH secretion by the pituitary can be suppressed. At 7:30 the next morning before eating I went to a medical lab to have blood samples drawn from my arm to measure my cortisol levels. It is important to do this test fasting first thing in the morning as cortisol levels change throughout the day and the mornings show more accurate levels.

Following the dexamethasone suppression test I was given an appointment for a growth hormone (GH) stimulation test at the hospital. During the GH stimulation test a special type of intravenous (IV) catheter would be inserted into a vein in my arm. A blood sample would be taken to measure pre-test blood levels of GH, glucose, and cortisol. Arginine (a basic protein amino acid), insulin (a hormone produced in the pancreas that regulates sugar), or GHRH (growth-hormone-releasing hormone) would then be infused through the IV line, blood samples would be obtained at several intervals over the course of two hours. I was monitored continuously for signs of hypoglycemia (weakness, restless-ness, hunger, sweating, and nervousness) and low blood pressure. I chewed ice chips to alleviate thirst.

When I went to the hospital for the GH stimulation test my husband and I were alarmed listening to people in the waiting room. Two women were talking about their chemotherapy treatments. They both had caps on because they obviously had lost their hair. They were joking about how it fell out. One lady said she plugged up her shower drain because it came out in such large clumps. They were talking like it was so normal and was just the way it was. They talked about how sick they would be in a couple of days after their chemo IVs that day and how they'd stay sick for another three or four days afterward. They were asking each other about their side effects. One of the women said by the time she was well enough to get out of bed it was time for another chemo treatment. The other responded, "I know what you mean," and recounted her problems with her blood levels being so low and had to get added shots to make her white blood counts increase. She also described all the sores she got in her mouth. They spoke so nonchalantly about all of it that it made me sick to my stomach.

As we sat and watched as people came in, some with walkers; one lady had an oxygen mask on and smelled like cigarettes. A man came in and sat down next to us. He looked like he was on his death bed. He told my husband that he was just healing from cancer surgery but while he was in the hospital he was exposed to MRSA, a bacterial infection that is often resistant to antibiotics. He said he almost died and now had to do chemotherapy. I thought, "Oh my god, how can the medical profession do this to people? How could they give chemotherapy to someone so sick?" I thought, "This man is not going to make it." My name was then called.

I was put in a room where cancer patients received their chemotherapy IVs. There were eight people in the room all sitting in reclining chairs, including me. The woman across from me was the woman who had come in with a walker and smelled liked cigarettes. She appeared to be older than me, but maybe she wasn't. She said she had a lung cancer recurrence and was there for her first round of chemotherapy since the recurrence. This would be her third round of chemotherapy since her diagnosis and surgery. And she's still smoking, I thought to myself.

A man on the other side of her received an IV of chemotherapy. He looked emaciated and could barely sit up in the chair, another "death-warmed-over-looking" person. It looked as if he had reached the point of accepting he wasn't going to live. I could see it in every feature of his body—his eyes, his face, the way he carried himself. It was heart-breaking.

I was seated next to a woman who was going through her third chemotherapy treatment for stage II breast cancer with one axillary lymph node that tested cancerous. While I was waiting for my GH stimulation test she said she couldn't use her left arm anymore due to lymphedema, swelling caused by a blockage in the lymphatic system. It was wrapped and in a sling, rendering it useless. I was speechless and turned my head away to hide my shocked expression. When I turned to face her again she went on to describe all the problems and side effects she had from chemotherapy treatments. She wanted to talk about everything and I could tell she wanted me to ask her questions or comment on what she was saying. I couldn't comment right away. Finally, I asked her what kind of breast cancer she had. She said she didn't know, just stage

II. She was upset because her doctors took lymph nodes out, which caused lymphedema. She said at times it really hurt. She then paused, thinking about my question, and said in a very upsetting tone, "I don't know, it was breast cancer, isn't that enough?" She looked away from me toward her son who was there with her. I felt sorry for her. When she turned back to look at me I asked her what kind of chemo they were giving her. She didn't know that either and said it took a couple of hours just sitting there watching it go into her arm. Sometimes she got sick and sometimes she was okay and would fall asleep during the treatments. She said she still had two more treatments, but then had to do radiation following the chemo.

By this time the nurse had arrived to administer the GH stimulation IV. While it was being administered, the lady that was sitting next to me asked what I was doing there. I told her about the pituitary tumor and that I was getting an infusion that will tell how my pituitary gland was functioning. Then I told her I was still trying to decide about doing chemotherapy and radiation for my stage II triple negative breast cancer diagnosis. She told me, "Don't do it. It is the most hideous treatment ever and you are sick during the whole thing." She then pulled her cap off and said "Do you want to also look like this?" She had no hair and had sores on her head. I was horrified at what I was experiencing. I then told her I had researched some alternative cancer treatments that treat cancer without chemo. She got a tear in her eye and she wished she had done that. We stopped speaking to each other after that and I sat there for next three and a half hours reading during my IV and blood tests. After the GH stimulation test, I had an ACTH stimulation test.

During the ACTH stimulation test blood samples were drawn to record pre-test cortisol levels. Less than 30 minutes later, an ACTH analogue (cosyntropin, a synthetic hormone used to evaluate and diagnose cortisol disorders of the anterior pituitary gland) was injected into my arm, over a two-minute period. Blood samples were taken 30 and 60 minutes after the injection so they could be analyzed for cortisol levels in response to cosyntropin. This ACTH stimulation test measures how the adrenal glands *react* to the ACTH in the blood by measuring your body's cortisol levels. It's important not to confuse this test with an *ACTH test*, which simply measures the ACTH *levels* in your blood.

When I was done with my tests I called my husband to come and pick me up. On our way home I relayed all my observations and conversations from the day to my husband. While we discussed my experience, I couldn't help but think that all these people were going through chemotherapy as a matter of fact. They all spoke as if it was the only way to be cured of cancer and they were all willing to accept the side effects. I was astounded that most of them had no clue as to what kind of cancer they really had or what kind of chemotherapy they were undergoing. They all were there because their doctors told them to be there.

The following week after my tests, I received a call that my results were in and was given the earliest appointment to see my neurologist in March, 2012. I was nervous during my appointment but he soon put me at ease. He said some hormone levels were low but not below normal. The testosterone was the only hormone that may need attention. After this information was reviewed we discussed the surgery again and my neurologist agreed to wait for surgery. But we had to monitor the tumor with an MRI every three months.

Chapter Six

Proposed Chemotherapy and Radiation Treatment

GOING THROUGH PITUITARY TESTING helped me understand the effects of chemotherapy and radiation and ultimately helped me choose alternative treatments. My discovery about the effects of chemotherapy was a wakeup call! People who develop cancer need to do research to understand everything about chemotherapy drugs and their side effects. Too many times people just want a magic pill to cure them.

For those with cancer, it is important to know that the underlying principle of chemotherapy is to kill the cancer cells with chemicals that interfere with the process of cell division, either by damaging the proteins involved, or by damaging the cell's DNA itself. These chemicals cause the damaged, sick and well cells to commit suicide, which overtaxes the immune system. Mustard gas, if you can believe it, is now called nitrogen mustard and is used in chemotherapy. It works by physically modifying the DNA in the cells. By attacking the DNA, the drug prevents the cell from forming new cells.

Chemotherapy was discovered during World War II. Some soldiers who were accidentally exposed to mustard gas, used to poison enemy troops, were found to have developed toxic changes in their bone marrow cells that develop into blood cells. These changes caused low white blood cell counts. It was believed that since white blood cells and cancer cells both grow very rapidly, the doctors hypothesized that if mustard gas could destroy normal white blood cells, it seemed likely that it could also destroy cancerous ones. Two doctors at Yale University, Louis Goodman and Alfred Gilman, were recruited by the United States Department of Defense to investigate potential therapeutic applications of chemical warfare agents. In the course of that work, Goodman and Gilman observed that mustard gas was too volatile an agent to be suitable for laboratory experiments and developed a compound called *nitrogen mustard* which was studied and found to work against a cancer of the lymph nodes called lymphoma (lymphoma is a cancer of the white blood cells). Some patients with advanced lymphomas were given a form of this mustard gas intravenously. This agent served as the model for a long series of similar but more effective agents called alkylating agents that killed rapidly growing cancer cells by damaging their DNA.

Nitrogen mustard drugs are extremely toxic. In fact, they can actually cause cancer. Medical personnel who prepare these medications must wear protective garb such as gloves and avoid inhaling the powder. According to Drugs.com, treatment with Mustargen, one such mustard drug, can result in a patient developing a second malignant tumor. The International Agency for Research on Cancer calls it a "probable carcinogen," or cancer-causing agent.

Treating some cancers also involves hormone therapy. In 1878 Thomas Beatson discovered that the breasts of rabbits stopped producing milk after he removed ovaries. Because the idea that breasts were "held in control" by the ovaries, Beatson performed a test to remove the ovaries (called oophorectomy) in advanced breast cancer patients. He found that an oophorectomy often resulted in improvement for breast cancer patients. He also suspected that the ovaries may be the cause of carcinoma of the breast. He had discovered the stimulating effect of the female ovarian hormone (estrogen) on breast cancer, even before the hormone itself was discovered. Later scientists identified that dramatic regression of metastatic prostate cancer following removal of the testes. How hormones influence growth of cancer has guided its progress in developing as well as reducing the risk of breast and prostate cancers. Beatson was a pioneer in the field of oncology and has been called the "father" of endocrine ablation in cancer management. His work provided the foundation for understanding the role of estrogen on breast, ovarian and other malignant tumors and the modern use of anti-hormone therapy, such as tamoxifen to treat or prevent breast cancer. Tamoxifen blocks the actions of estrogen, a female hormone. Certain types of breast cancer require estrogen to grow.

Tamoxifen is a form of a chemo drug and taking tamoxifen increases the risk of getting cancer of the uterus (also called endometrial cancer), stokes and blood clotting problems. Tamoxifen has been used for more than thirty years to treat hormone receptor-positive breast cancer. My diagnosis TNBC does not respond to hormonal therapy such as tamoxifen or aromatase inhibitors or therapies that target hormone receptors so I am happy this treatment was not recommended for me.

Much of the chemotherapy today has not changed since the early 1960s. However, the applications of chemo drugs were applied in conjunction with surgery and/or radiation, initially in breast cancer patients. Radiation was used after surgery to control small tumor growths that were not surgically removed. Finally, chemotherapy was added to destroy small tumor growths that had spread beyond the reach of the surgeon and radiotherapist. Chemotherapy was then used after surgery to destroy any remaining cancer cells in the body or rogue cancer cells left in the body. New combinations of chemotherapy drugs and new delivery techniques were then implemented —adjuvant chemotherapy was born.

Patients receiving chemotherapy are at risk for developing infections that may lead to hospitalization, and even death. Chemotherapy treatments do not guarantee that the patient will be cured or that cancer won't come back. But doctors often try to prevent it from recurring anyway, as in my case. Sometimes only months later, the patient discovers that the cancer is back and more aggressive than it was the first time. This is because the immune system has been so damaged by the chemo drugs it cannot fight back.

Unfortunately, as a society, we have been trained to blindly believe in the traditional medical system. For example, after receiving only the "standard" conventional treatment, cancer patients often believe that they are cured because their cancer is in remission. Remarkably in December 2004 a groundbreaking fourteen year study was published in the Journal of Clinical Oncology called "The Contribution of Cytotoxic Chemotherapy to 5-year Survival in Adult Malignancies". Researchers at the Department of Radiation Oncology at the Northern Sydney Cancer Centre studied the five-year survival rates of chemotherapy on twenty-two types of cancers in the United States and Australia. They studied 154,971 Americans and Australians with cancer, age twenty and older, which were treated with conventional treatments, including chemotherapy. Only 3,306 had survival that could be credited to chemotherapy. The study results were that the overall contribution of curative and adjuvant cytotoxic chemotherapy to five-year survival in adults was estimated to be 2.3% in Australia and 2.1 % in the United States. The fact that chemo only contributes on average about 2% to the overall survival rate is very alarming, and probably something doctors will not mention to a cancer patient. It certainly was not mentioned to me and Cytoxan was one of my recommended chemo drugs.

The following are the drugs that were recommended to me as the most aggressive form of therapy because I was stage II triple negative breast cancer. As discussed, TNBC has no receptors so targeted chemotherapies would not work; therefore my doctors felt that systemic adjunctive chemotherapy would be best.

Several chemotherapy treatments were recommended which included *Doxorubicin* chemotherapy. Its nickname is "red death or red evil" because the bodily fluids turn red during treatment. When I mentioned this fact to my oncologist, he scoffed and said he never heard of such a thing. My arguments with him and his negative reaction gave evidence to me that he did not want to admit what I found out to be true. Nor did he want me to be knowledgeable about chemotherapy treatments. He just wanted me to do it, period. I told my doctor that during my researching of the drug I learned it has been known to also cause congestive heart failure, which also frightened me. He responded by saying "Everything has side effects." I quit seeing my oncologist after that day.

Another drug therapy recommended to me was *Cytoxan*. It is classified as an "alkylating agent"—mustard gas. Yes, I said mustard gas! It is still used today. Other cytotoxic drugs related to cyclophosphamide (Cytoxan) are chlorambucil (Leukeran) and nitrogen mustard (Mustargen). Leukeran and Mustargen have had similar side effects as Cytoxan. These two drugs, Doxorubicin and Cytoxan, were to be given as adjuvant chemotherapy treatment following my surgery (injections every fourteen days consisting of eight cycles—four months). It would be a chemical "cocktail" so to speak.

After being administered the "cocktail," I would then receive another chemotherapy drug called *Paclitaxel* (injections every seven days for twelve weeks—three months). Paclitaxel is an anti-cancer Cytotoxic chemotherapy drug—mustard gas. This drug is typically used to treat breast cancer after the failure of the adjuvant chemotherapy "cocktail," within six months of having received adjuvant chemotherapy. (In other words, this chemo drug fixes what the other two chemotherapies couldn't fix, like keeping cancer from coming back.)

These three chemo drug side effects would have been nausea, vomiting, diarrhea, unusual bleeding or bruising, black or tarry stools, blood in the stools, and blood in the urine. How would someone know if bleeding occurs? A side effect of one of the drugs was red bodily fluid. Other side effects include pain or burning with urination, extreme fatigue (unable to carry on self-care activities), mouth sores (painful redness, swelling, or ulcers), congestive heart failure, loss of hair, the development of other cancers such as leukemia and/or bone cancer and much more.

After the chemotherapy treatments, I would receive twelve weeks (three months) of radiation therapy five days a week. Radiation therapy uses special equipment to send high doses of radiation to the cancer cells. Most cells in the body grow and divide to form new cells. But cancer cells grow and divide faster than many of the normal cells around them. Radiation works by making small breaks in the DNA inside cells. Sometimes radiation is given at the same time as the chemotherapy, but not in my case. Even radiation has side effects but doctors say "they're not bad." According to the National Cancer Institute, many people who receive radiation therapy do have side effects. Skin changes may include dryness, itching, peeling, or blistering. These changes occur because radiation therapy damages healthy skin cells in the treatment area. Most patients often experience fatigue, feeling extremely worn out or exhausted. Other potential side effects may also include diarrhea, hair loss in the treatment area, mouth sores, nausea and vomiting, swelling, problems swallowing and urinary and bladder changes. Sexual change can occur for some cancer patients such as an overall loss of desire. For men, erection problems are a common problem. For women, vaginal dryness and pain with sexual activity are frequent. Most of these side effects go away within two months after radiation therapy is finished. Late side effects may occur six or more months after radiation therapy ends. These effects may include infertility, joint problems, lymphedema, mouth sores, and other secondary cancers.

The Mayo Clinic documented that acute myelogenous leukemia (AML), chronic myelogenous leukemia (CML), and acute lymphoblastic leukemia (ALL) have been linked to radiation exposure. Myelodysplastic syndrome (MDS), a bone marrow disorder that can turn into acute leukemia, has also been linked to radiation exposure.

The risk of these diseases after radiation treatment depends on a number of factors such as, how much of the body's bone marrow was exposed to radiation, the amount of radiation that reached active bone marrow and the radiation dose rate (how much was given in each dose, how long it took to give the dose, and how often it was given).

The person's age when they were treated with radiation does not seem to be a risk factor. Most cases usually develop within several years of radiation treatment, peaking at five to nine years after exposure. Then the number of cases developing slowly declines over the following years. Some cancers require larger doses of radiation than others, and certain treatment techniques use more radiation. The area treated is also important as cancers tend to develop in or near the area that was treated with radiation. Certain organs, such as the breast and thyroid, seem to be more likely to develop cancers after radiation than others.

The American Cancer Society indicates that other cancers, which are mostly solid tumors, have been shown to take much longer to develop. "Most of these cancers are not seen for at least ten years after radiation therapy, and some are diagnosed even more than fifteen years later. The effect of radiation on the risk of developing a solid tumor cancer depends on such factors as the dose of radiation, the area treated, and the age of the patient when treated with radiation.

In general, the risk of developing a solid tumor after radiation treatment goes up as the dose of radiation increases. Some cancers require larger doses of radiation than others, and certain techniques require more radiation. For example, intensity modulated radiation therapy (IMRT), delivers precise radiation doses to a malignant tumor or specific areas within the tumor. It also helps to protect tissues that are more easily injured by radiation, but a larger dose of radiation overall must be used."[1]

Radiation has been used in many ways and in many forms since it was first discovered in the late 1800s. In 1896 a German physics professor, Wilhelm Conrad Roentgen, presented a remarkable lecture titled "Concerning a New Kind of Ray." Roentgen called it the "X-ray", with "x" being the algebraic symbol for an unknown quantity. Nearly two weeks after his discovery, he took the very first picture using X-rays of his wife Anna Bertha's hand which produced a skeleton picture. This caused such great excitement that within months, systems were being designed to use X-rays machines.

Henri Becquerel, a French physicist, announced a similar discovery of penetrating rays emitted from salts of uranium. However, it did not draw as much attention as X-rays. This led to a breakthrough in France with the discovery that daily doses of radiation over several weeks improved a patient's chance for a cancer cure. Within three years after this discovery radiation was used to treat cancer. X-ray machines were being used for diagnosis as well as therapy.

In the early 1900s, experimenters and physicians subjected their hands and skin to an X-ray for half an hour each day for several days. The effects were pain, swelling, stiffness, erythema (sunburn like redness) and blistering skin. These experiments were later called the "erythema dose," and this was considered an estimate of the proper daily radiation doses. These experiments led to another discovery that radiation could cause cancer as well as cure it as many experimenters and physicians developed leukemia from regularly exposing themselves to radiation.

Up to 10% of invasive cancers are related to radiation exposure. Ionizing radiation can cause changes in the chemical balance of cells and some of those changes can result in cancer. In addition, by damaging the genetic material (DNA) contained in all cells of the body, ionizing radiation can cause harmful genetic mutations that can be passed on to future generations.

"Advances in radiation physics and computer technology during the last quarter of the 20th century made it possible to aim radiation more precisely. *Conformal radiation therapy (CRT)* uses CT images and special computers to very precisely map the location of a cancer in three dimensions. A patient is fitted with a plastic mold or cast to keep the body part still and in the same position for each treatment. The radiation beams are matched to the shape of the tumor and delivered to the tumor from several directions.

Intensity-modulated radiation therapy (IMRT) is like CRT, but along with aiming photon-beam radiation from several directions, the intensity (strength) of the beams can be adjusted. This therapy gives doctors even more control by decreasing the radiation reaching normal tissue while delivering a high dose to the cancer cell.

A related technique, *conformal proton beam radiation therapy*, uses a similar approach to focusing radiation on the cancer. But instead of using X-rays, this technique uses proton beams. Protons are parts of atoms that cause little damage to tissues they pass through but are very effective in killing cells at the end of their path. This means that proton beam radiation can deliver more radiation to the cancer while possibly reducing damage to nearby normal tissues.

Stereotactic radiosurgery and *stereotactic radiation therapy* are terms that describe several techniques used to deliver a large, precise radiation dose to a small tumor. The term *surgery* may be confusing because no cutting is actually done. The most common site treated with this radiation technique is the brain.

Intraoperative radiation therapy (IORT) is a form of treatment that delivers radiation at the time of surgery. The radiation can be given directly to the cancer or to the nearby tissues after the cancer has been removed. It's most commonly used in abdominal or pelvic cancers and in cancers that tend to recur. IORT minimizes the amount of tissue that's exposed to radiation because normal tissues can be moved out of the way during surgery and shielded, allowing a higher dose of radiation to be directed at the cancer.

Chemical modifiers or *radio sensitizers* are substances that make cancer more sensitive to radiation. The goal of research into these types of substances is to develop agents that will make the tumor more sensitive without affecting normal tissues. Researchers are also looking for substances that may help protect normal cells from radiation." [2]

Despite all of these advances in radiation therapy—radiation was still a problem as far as I was concerned!

In my case with TNBC, clinical trials indicated that chemotherapy would only have added 12% to my life expectancy due to TNBC's rapid growth and its invasive nature. The arduous treatments would last almost a year. I would have needed help as I would be sick and unable to get out of bed most of the time. I wouldn't be able to shave my legs or arm-pits with a razor when my hair grew back as I might cut myself and bleeding could be a problem. I would have to wear a mask if I went out in public and no friends or family members could come to our house if they were sick because my immune system would be too compromised and I could be hospitalized if I got their illness. With all this infor-mation, one question pervaded my thoughts: "Do I really want or need chemotherapy or radiation?"

Chapter Seven

Researching Alternative Treatments

WHILE I WAS RESEARCHING MY pituitary situation and my chemotherapy cancer concerns, I came across the idea that we need to look at the underlying causes of cancer—not "mask" the problem using chemotherapy to respond to the symptoms. I learned that alternative cancer treatments help the body fight off the recurring cancer cells by boosting the immune system. Boosting the immune system is particularly important during chemotherapy treatments. These types of treatments can provide cancer patients the best chance of staying cancer free long term. Every human being has cancer cells. The body's natural defense identifies and destroys them before they become tumors. My thought was that my body is making tumors so I need to find and correct my underlying problem.

Dr. Parviz Ghadirian at the University of Montreal studied women who carried the BRAC1 and BRAC2 genes. He discovered that the more fruits and vegetables these at-risk women ate per week their cancer risk diminished by 73%. It is now recommended to eat five or more servings of a variety of fruits and vegetables each day. Professor John Witte of the

University of San Francisco made a similar discovery in men with prostate cancer. Consuming oily, omega-3 rich fish at least twice a week, kept prostate cancer in check, specifically eating dark fish such as salmon. And the prostate cancers in those men were five times less likely to become aggressive than in those men that did not eat omega-3 oily fish at all.

During my research I discovered metabolic therapy. Metabolic therapy uses a combination of special diets, enzymes, nutritional supplements, and other measures in an attempt to remove "toxins" from the body and strengthen the body's defenses against disease. Toxic substances in food and the environment build up in the body and create chemical imbalances that lead to diseases such as cancer, arthritis, and multiple sclerosis. Metabolic therapy aims to rid the body of these toxins and strengthens its resistance to disease. With special diet serious illnesses, including cancer can be cured.

Metabolic therapies vary a great deal depending on the practitioner, but all are based on special diets and detoxification. They usually incorporate natural, whole foods such as fresh fruits and vegetables, as well as vitamins and mineral supplements. Other measures may include colonics, coffee enemas, juicing, enzyme supplements, visualization, and stress-reduction exercises. Among the better known types of metabolic therapy are the Kelley Metabolic treatment, the Gonzalez Regimen treatment, Issels whole body therapy, and the Gerson Therapy. There are many more metabolic therapies, however, these are the ones I researched and know.

The Kelley metabolic treatment was developed in the 1960s by American orthodontist William Donald Kelley, DDS, MS. It includes dietary supplements (such as enzymes and large doses of vitamins, minerals, and amino acids), detoxification (such as fasting, exercising, and using laxatives and coffee enemas), a restricted diet, chiropractic adjustments, and prayer. Dr. Kelley held that a root cause of cancer is the body's inability to metabolize (digest and utilize) protein. If the protein metabolism is not corrected, the body has more tumors in the future, even if the first one is successfully removed. Unfortunately this is the reason why so many successful cancer operations end up in recurrences a year or two later. The tumor was removed but the cause, improper protein metabolism, remained. Practitioners classify people into different metabolic types which form the individual dietary and supplement recommendations.

Nicholas Gonzalez, MD, became interested in metabolic therapy as a medical student in 1981 when he was asked to review Dr. Kelley's work. He became inspired to develop his own therapy. The Gonzalez is similar to Kelley's treatment but it includes extracts such as thymus and liver and digestive enzymes as part of the plan. The regimen can be broken down into the following basic components: diet, supplements (with pancreas product for cancer patients), and detoxification routines such as coffee enemas. Although most of the published research about the Gonzalez treatment deals with pancreatic cancer, it is used to treat patients with all types of cancers and also treat patients with a variety of other problems, ranging from chronic fatigue syndrome to multiple sclerosis. The treatment is individualized for each patient.

Another form of metabolic therapy is Issels whole body therapy. Patients using this therapy are asked to remove fillings that contain mercury, follow a strict diet, and eliminate the use of tobacco, coffee, tea, and other substances that are considered harmful. Some patients are encouraged to relieve stress and deal with anger and emotional distress. Issels Integrative Immuno-Oncology therapy has two lines of approach and each is of equal importance: therapies specific to the cancer cells and tumors, such as non-toxic cancer vaccines and cell therapies, and gene-targeted cancer therapies and personalized standard cancer treatment protocols, including non-toxic immunobiologic core treatment to alter the tumor microenvironment, which plays a pivotal role in cancer progression or regression and healing. The program is a treatment that is applicable for types and all stages of cancer.

The Gerson Therapy involves a strict dietary program and is similar to the Kelley and Gonzalez therapies. The Gerson Therapy aims to bring

the body back to health, supporting each important metabolic require-
ment by flooding the body daily with nutrients from organically-grown
fruits and vegetables. Most is used to make fresh raw juice. Raw and
cooked solid fruits and vegetables are generously consumed. Eating large
volumes of these foods usually more than doubled the amount of oxygen
in the blood, as oxygen deficiency contributes to many degenerative
diseases. The metabolism is also stimulated through the addition of
thyroid, potassium, and other supplements. Patients avoid heavy animal
fats, excess protein, sodium, and other toxins. The Gerson Therapy uses
intensive detoxification to eliminate wastes, regenerate the liver,
reactivate the immune system, and restore the body's enzymes, minerals
and hormones—the body's essential defense systems.

There are many other alternative programs out there similar to the
Gerson Therapy that are also very good programs. German biochemist
and author Johanna Budwig was a pharmacist and held doctorate degrees
in physics and chemistry. Based on her research on fatty acids on 1952,
she developed a diet that she believed was useful in the treatment of
cancer. The diet is based on modifying dietary fats. It is rich in flaxseed
oil, often mixed with cottage cheese, and meals high in fruits, vegetables,
and fiber. The diet recommends avoiding sugar, animal fats, salad oil,
meats, butter, and especially margarine.

In the 1970s and 1980s, biology professor Harold Manner, PhD, was
also a major proponent of metabolic therapy. In Dr. Manner's book *The
Death of Cancer* claims cancer can be controlled through nutritional
guidance, a positive attitude, and changes in lifestyle. His metabolic
program includes the use of natural foods, lessons in the preparation of a
"low-stress" diet, enzyme and vitamin therapy, fasting, and coffee
enemas.   He has cured cancer in mice with injections of laetrile,
enzymes, and vitamin A. In his version of metabolic cancer therapy,
patients often receive another alternative substance, a chemical
compound called dimethyl sulfoxide (DMSO) to relieve pain and swelling in musculoskeletal disorders.

The more I researched alternative treatments and the more I thought about chemotherapy and all the side effects, I started to reverse my thoughts about what I would do. I began to tell the doctors I already did the "cut" part and didn't want the "poison and burn" part of the therapy. I argued that I would die first by the chemotherapy itself if not by cancer in a year. All this did was make everyone upset, including me. In my mind, to them, I was only a statistic and statistics are the norm. I am not the norm! And with my new found knowledge, I figured why should I die? I wanted to be as healthy as I could, be happy and have the best quality of life I could with my husband, children, grandchildren, and all my family and friends for the rest of whatever life I had left. I came to the same conclusion that David Servan-Schreiber, MD & PHD did in his book, *Anti Cancer A New Way of Life* that if I had not been diagnosed with cancer, I would not have known how unhealthy my lifestyle truly was.

My husband, children and I continued researching alternative therapies. We went to book stores and kept coming across the same book again and again *Healing the Gerson Way: Defeating Cancer and Other Chronic Diseases* by Charlotte Gerson and Beata Bishop. My oldest son found the same information on Gerson. Our son's friend also found the same information while he was researching alternative cancer approaches. Information abounded! We were all amazed that we came to the same conclusion. We felt we were led to this book and ordered it.

Ultimately, I chose NOT to do chemotherapy or radiation and chose an alternative approach to treat my cancer. I chose the Gerson Therapy, not just a diet developed by Dr. Max Gerson but a lifestyle change.

The doctors tried to convince me that chemotherapy was the answer. I had listened to all their recommendations and had thoroughly done my research. Everything became clear to me and it all made sense. I needed to be healthier, not poison my body. I needed to shed old ideas, habits, and opinions. I had to let go, which was a very difficult decision.

I believe that all people have the ability to change their lives. They just need to make it their own decision. Research will reveal what lifestyle change is best for each individual.

There has been a lot of skepticism about alternative treatments that heal by using herbs, vitamins, and nutrition. They have been called all kinds of things, such as charlatan and shyster programs. Many opponents to these programs say that relying on these treatments alone and avoiding or delaying conventional medical care may have serious health consequences because there is no "scientific" evidence to prove otherwise. I would suggest the same is true for chemotherapy and that perhaps the death rate from traditional cancer treatments is much higher than what is being reported.

During traditional cancer treatments, the DNA cell is altered or damaged and both good and bad cells die. The immune system is practically nonexistent and cancer cells can eventually become resistant to the chemo drugs. Cancer comes back with vengeance. Traditional cancer treatments probably cause cancer patients to die earlier or render them incurable because the chemo drugs that were originally administered couldn't fix or keep cancer from coming back.

The fact that thousands of people, all over the world, are living a healthy life after completing an alternative treatment was evidence for me, "scientific" or not. Cancer patients going through alternative treatments often have a much better quality of life than patients going through chemotherapy or radiation. They are still alive and I am one of them.

Part II

Alternative Treatment, The Experience, and
The Importance of Testing and Monitoring
Health

Chapter Eight

The Gerson Therapy, The Treatment

YES, I CHOSE THE GERSON THERAPY. It has been documented that this treatment achieved a true cure rate of 50% on advanced terminal patients, which is exceptional because he counted all of his patients, not just those who lived for a year or more. Conventional medicine is just now agreeing that nutrition is an essential part of healing. Albeit Dr. Max Gerson's treatment is very complex as well as his book, but it does have merit and common sense. During the time he was practicing medicine the cancer patients that were sent home to die were in better health than the cancer patients that are sent home to die today. His book *A Cancer Therapy: Results of Fifty Cases and the Cure of Advanced Cancer by Diet Therapy 6th Edition* is quite long and very technical. But I recommend reading it, especially for those using his treatment.

During my research I came across several documentary films, which I have referenced at the end of my book. One film stood out to me most by filmmaker Stephen Kroschel, *The Beautiful Truth*. Mr. Kroschel wanted to find hard evidence of the effectiveness of natural cancer treatment claimed by the Gerson Therapy. He travelled across the Atlantic and Pacific Oceans, Japan, Holland and Mexico and many parts of the United States. At the end of the film, he has testimonies of patients, scientists, surgeons and nutritionists, who testify the effectiveness of the Gerson Therapy and shows the hard scientific evidence to back up their claims. It is an informative and a stimulating documentary. He reveals the cover-ups in the health industry and the censorship of cures for many diseases and ailments, including cancer. I was deeply moved and it helped convince me I was on the right track to do the Gerson Therapy.

Dr. Gerson was born in Wongrowitz (Wagrowiec, now in Poland), on October 18, 1881. In 1909, he graduated from the Albert-Ludwigs Universität Freiburg. He began practicing medicine at age 28 in Breslau (Wroclaw, now in Poland), later specializing in internal medicine and nerve diseases. By 1927, he specialized in the treatment of tuberculosis, developing the Gerson-Sauerbruch-Hermannsdorfer diet. Dr. Max Gerson did not set out to cure cancer. Initially it was a treatment for his debilitating migraines and after developing a diet that alleviated his headaches, he recommended his diet to his patients who suffered from migraines. One of his patients not only recovered from migraines but his skin tuberculosis healed as well. Dr. Gerson then tried his therapy on cancer patients in 1928. Through his work he attracted the friendship of Dr. Albert Schweitzer. In 1931 after nine months of applying Dr. Gerson's therapy on Dr. Schweitzer's wife, Helene Bresslau-Schweitzer, was cured of lung tuberculosis. Dr. Schweitzer himself was cured of his advanced adult diabetes after only a few weeks applying Dr. Gerson's therapy and was completely off his heavy insulin dosage. Over the years, Dr. Gerson refined his diet and detoxification therapy, concentrating on eradicating cancer. He later moved to the United States, settling in New York City where he passed his medical board examination and became a U.S. citizen in 1942.

Dr. Gerson's daughter, Charlotte Gerson, founded the Gerson Insti-tute in 1977, to spread awareness of the Gerson Therapy and make it available to people across the world. The Gerson Institute is a non-profit organization located in San Diego, California, dedicated to providing education and training in the Gerson Therapy. It promotes the alternative, nontoxic treatment program for cancer and other chronic degenerative diseases in the same manner that Max Gerson had intended almost sixty years ago.

How does the therapy work?

The diet is naturally high in vitamins, minerals, enzymes, micronutrients and is extremely low in sodium and fats. The therapy activates the body's extraordinary ability to heal itself through an organic, vegetarian diet, raw juices, coffee enemas and natural supplements. The therapy treats the underlying causes of disease: toxicity and nutritional deficiency. It is a non-specific treatment that effectively treats many different conditions by healing the body as a whole, rather than selectively targeting a specific condition or symptom. Over the past 60 years, thousands of people have used the Gerson Therapy to recover from so-called incurable diseases and I am one of them.

The Gerson diet is plant-based and entirely organic. It has an abundance of nutrients from large amounts of fresh, organic juices that are consumed every day which provide the body with enzymes, minerals and nutrients. The following is a typical daily diet for a Gerson patient on the full therapy regimen:

- Thirteen glasses of fresh, raw carrot/apple and green-leaf juices prepared hourly from fresh, organic fruits, and vegetables.
- Three full plant-based meals, freshly prepared from organically grown fruits, vegetables and whole grains. A typical meal could include salad, cooked vegetables, baked potatoes, soup, and juice.
- Fresh fruit and vegetables for snacks, in addition to the regular diet.[1]

All medications used by patients in connection with the Gerson Therapy are classed as biological materials of organic origin. They are supplied in therapeutic amounts for healing and to prevent overdosing. The most used supplements as a part of the Gerson Therapy include:

- Potassium compound (replenishes electrolytes)
- Lugol's solution (corrects iodine deficiency, detoxifies heavy metals, and assists the thyroid)
- Vitamin B12 (increases blood flow and when vitamin B12, folic acid, and vitamin C are used together it has been shown to help protect memory and thinking skills)
- Pancreatic enzymes (helps the pancreas break down fats, proteins, and carbohydrates)
- Liver supplements (helps assist the liver eliminate potentially toxic chemicals)

On the Gerson Therapy, coffee enemas are the primary method of detoxifying the body's tissues and blood. An enema is the introduction of a solution into the rectum and colon in order to stimulate bowel activity, causing the lower intestine to be emptied.

The content of the large intestine is the biggest blood poisoning source, which also poisons the liver and other vital organs thereby being important to cleanse. When cleansing the large intestine (colon), fecal stones are eliminated (result of the wrong food combining). Cleansing also eliminates toxic mucus and bile, parasites, mucoid plaque (rubber-like strings), which is a result of poisonous intestinal "plants" and thriving parasites. Cancer patients on the Gerson Therapy may take up to five coffee enemas each day. Charlotte Gerson describes the importance of flushing the system: "The moment a patient is put on the full therapy, the combined effect of the food, the juices and the medication causes the immune system to attack and kill tumor tissue, besides working to flush out accumulated toxins from the body tissues. This great clearing-out procedure carries the risk of overburdening and poisoning the liver, the all-important organ of detoxification, which in a cancer patient is, bound to be already damaged and debilitated." [2]

I read John Gunther's *Death Be Not Proud* and I quote him regarding his thoughts on Gerson because I am in total agreement: "The Gerson diet is saltless and fatless, and for a long time proteins are excluded or held to an extreme minimum. The theory behind this is simple enough. Give nature opportunity, and nature herself will heal. It is the silliest thing in the world to attempt to arrest cancer of the tongue, say, but cutting off the tongue. What the physician should strive for, if he gets a case in time, is to change the metabolism of the body so that the cancer (or another affliction) dies of itself. The whole theory is erected on the basis that the chemistry of the body can be so altered as to eliminate disease."[3]

To best implement the Gerson Therapy in my life I decided to attend an intensive therapy training session at a center. I attended The Longevity Center (TLC), a Redlands, California facility along with my husband and caretaker, John. There we learned and experienced the incredible healing power of nutrition and coffee enemas, which is based on the work of Dr. Max Gerson. The Gerson Therapy is an extremely complex and comprehensive treatment, and taking it all in at once can be overwhelming. When classes are taught about the Gerson Therapy, it is broken down into bite-sized pieces to make it easier for people to learn and remember everything.

At TLC we learned the importance of adhering to the strict dietary guidelines and how changes without the advice of a certified Gerson Therapy practitioner could be harmful. Too many "minor modifications" to the Gerson Therapy protocol could impede the healing process. The Gerson Therapy has been shown to be successful in achieving remission and curing many different diseases when it is used as directed. We learned about cancer fighting foods, desirable foods, accepted spices, oils and sweeteners, and prohibited foods, which were practically drilled into us. We could occasionally have other allowed foods such as whole rye breads once a day, sweeteners like pure maple syrup, honey, unrefined blackstrap molasses could be used sparingly once a day, brown or wild rice once a week, yams, sweet potatoes and bananas once a week and even organic popcorn but as a holiday treat only.

Our stay at the center lasted ten days and was an intensive training session. All our meals, supplements, and room and lodging were included. When the clinic is over the patient goes home to complete the program on their own. Cancer patients are committed to the program for two years. The disease will determine the program length. Some patients just use the program as a maintenance program or life style change. The patient is encouraged to keep in contact with the Gerson practitioner. I was in constant contact with my practitioner after we went home during the entire two year program. I could call, text or email any concerns or question I might have. My conventional doctors' reports and blood tests were forwarded to my practitioner. If he saw things which triggered concerns, he would discuss them with me and corrections were made regarding meals or supplements. I stayed in contact with him; first weekly, then gradually monthly when I became more comfortable and "owned" the program. Even though I have finished my two year protocol, I still request advise every once in awhile and it is gladly given.

Attending the clinic is important! We learned the dos and don'ts about cooking food, the proper way to juice, the value of all the supplements and why they are so important to the program. Reading the book without the actual in-person teachings of the program could limit a patient's ability to fully heal. We read the book but to have the hands on experience learning the proper way to juice and eat was far more illuminating than reading alone.

Before I attended The Longevity Center, I did not want to do the coffee enemas, which I felt was the most bizarre part of the therapy. My husband and I argued about it and finally I relinquished when we went to the center. The coffee enema is, without a doubt, the most unusual part of Gerson's regime, and many are astonished by it, including me. However, the coffee enema has a very specific purpose: lowering serum toxins. Without the enemas, the program could not be at its optimum.

It is also important to mention that when doing coffee enemas common sense must be used. The coffee should be at room temperature or lukewarm to prevent burning the rectum. There have been cases of people who did not use caution while administering the enemas, which fed the frenzy that the therapy is bad or dangerous. A common sense approach should be used no matter what treatment is invoked—whether it is conventional or alternative treatment.

Lee W. Wattenberg and coworkers of the Department of Laboratory Medicine and Pathology at the University of Minnesota were able to prove in 1981 that the palmitic acid (fatty acids) found in green coffee beans promotes the activity of a key enzyme system called glutathione-S-transferase (GSH). GSH is the most powerful antioxidant which is a chemical that blocks the activity of other chemicals known as free radicals. GSH in green coffee beans increases by multiple times above the norm (between 78 and 182%) and neutralizes free radicals, unstable atoms that can damage cells. Instant coffee had 50% less GSH and was not as effective. GSH is a major detoxification enzyme system. Glutathione absorbs free radicals and renders them inert. Once they have been absorbed into bile, free radicals become dissolved matter and are eliminated from the body. When cells are challenged by poison, oxygen starvation, malnutrition, or trauma, a uniform set of reactions takes place: cells lose potassium, accept excess sodium and chloride, and swell with excess water. The palmitic acid from the coffee enemas, act as a powerful force to help rid the body of these toxic cells.

Dr. Peter Lechner, an oncologist and surgeon at the District Hospital in Graz, Austria, uses coffee enemas in the hospital's post-surgery programs. His decision to incorporate coffee enemas is based on experimental research done at the University of Minnesota, using the Gonzalez Regimen I described earlier. His research has demonstrated the beneficial effects of alkaloids (a class of nitrogenous organic compounds of plant origin that have pronounced physiological actions on humans) and palmiates (fatty acids). However, the US Food and Drug Administration (FDA) has not approved the Gonzalez Regimen or the Gerson Therapy or any other cancer treatments such as these. Of course not! Food cannot be patented like drugs and the drug industry is huge in lobbying the FDA. Drugs equal money!

With all the new found knowledge from the clinic, we returned home and cleaned out our pantry and filled it with only organic products. We had an extra refrigerator in the shed and moved it into the house for all the vegetables and fruit needed for juicing. We already had good stainless steel cookware but we bought other essentials, such as a plethora of glassware for food storage and a better juicer.

Obtaining the best juices for green vegetables required a masticating juicer, versus an extraction juicer. An extraction juicer uses centrifugal force and work best with soft and hard fruits and vegetables, but not with leafy greens like kale, lettuce, spinach, or with wheatgrass and tends to have more product waste. Masticating juicers, typically have a horizontal design, such as the Champion, our first juicer. The masticating juicers tube contains an auger that extends out of the motorized base and grinds the food to soften or reduce it to pulp, which produces more juice than a centrifugal juicer. We later chose the Norwalk masticating juicer with a vertical auger because it had a built in hydraulic press. After the food is reduced to pulp it is pressed to release the juice and utilizes much more of the product and better juice. We discovered it was much easier to clean, especially since we were juicing ten to thirteen juices a day. The Norwalk ranges from $1,600 used to $2,500 new. However, we still use our Champion juicer to take with us on trips as it is smaller. The Champion ranges from $100 used and $350 new. We take juicing very seriously and feel the expense is worth our health.

During the clinic we also learned about cleaning products and how toxic many of them can be in our home environment. The very first thing we did when we came home from the clinic was to hire a cleaning company to clean our home from top to bottom (similar to spring cleaning), including all the windows, using only natural or biodegradable cleaners. We discarded all chemical cleaners from the house and replaced them only with natural or biodegradable cleansers.

We no longer use air fresheners or aerosols. Instead, we simmer a pot of water on the stove with herbs or pure essential oils for fragrance as commercial air fresheners mask smells and can coat nasal passages to diminish the sense of smell. Aerosols, particularly insect repellents, are loaded with poisons. Therefore, we make our own natural insect repellent by mixing a few drops of tea tree oil with coconut oil in a spray bottle. The strong smell of tea tree oil naturally repels insects and the coconut oil absorbs very well on the skin, shrubbery and plants outside the house. A drop of tee tree oil on the skin is great for relieving the itch from insect bites and is also a fantastic antiseptic. For other skin conditions we simply apply a few drops of oil to minor cuts, burns, and infections. Adding a few drops of this oil during the wash cycle makes our laundry smell crisper and kill organisms lurking in the washer. Baking soda is another inexpensive way to clean and deodorize and using it with tee tree oil makes it even better. Simply mix a half cup baking soda and about 20 drops tea tree oil in a cup and sprinkle it on the carpets. After fifteen minutes it can be vacuumed and the home smells clean and fresh.

BonAmi is a biodegradable cleaning agent that is made from limestone, feldspar, coconut and corn husks and has baking soda as an ingredient. I find it is the best cleanser for heavy duty jobs in the bathroom, kitchen and pots and pans. For lighter pots and pan jobs olive oil can be used sparingly to clean stainless steel with a scouring pad.

White distilled vinegar is an inexpensive product with many uses. It will cut grease, remove mildew, odor, some stains and wax build-up. We apply a little vinegar and olive oil on a rag and use that for dusting our wood furniture and surfaces in lieu of store bought polishes. We also use vinegar as a fabric softener. Fabric softeners can cause asthma problems so we use a quarter cup of distilled vinegar in the laundry instead. Cornstarch can be used to clean windows by making it into a soft paste then rinse them with water and white distilled vinegar. Voila! Clean windows.

We use hydrogen peroxide in lieu of chlorine and biodegradable flakes or powders for our laundry. Hydrogen peroxide is also wonderful cleaning the kitchen or bathroom as well as isopropyl alcohol which is also an excellent disinfectant. Lemons are one of the strongest food-acids, effective against most household bacteria. We use it to wipe down bread boards after they are cleaned with water and a mild soap. The soap we use in liquid form is Castile which is excellent for dishes, bathing and lightly cleaning floors. However, Simple Green is an effective, non-toxic, non-flammable, biodegradable and non-abrasive general house hold cleaner and works well on our floors very well.

I am pleased I am able to share the few things we have learned to do to keep our household safe from toxic influences. Keep aware of your surroundings and discover the best way to keep your environment safe.

Chapter Nine

A Day in the Life of Treatment,
The Experience

WHEN WE FIRST STARTED THE PROGRAM on our own, I was defiant. Dealing with cancer and making a lifestyle change was overwhelming. It was emotionally draining. I cried and argued. But once I got on board and realized I was facing death, I made the change and I never looked back. My husband is some kind of a saint to have put up with all my moods.

The Gerson Therapy is difficult until it becomes routine. Establishing a routine for the amount of time spent juicing and preparing food definitely requires an assistant or a caregiver. The caregiver must be willing to be involved, doesn't mind being in the kitchen, and is able to stay home with you until you are strong enough to take over. My husband and I are not wealthy people so we decided together that he could be my caregiver. We both took early retirement which turned out to be a good thing. We worked hard all our lives, made good decisions regarding a 401k and pension plans, and now have social security. We have learned to be frugal, but not cheap. We are fortunate to live a decent comfortable life within our means.

My first three month Gerson Therapy was very difficult until we got the hang of it. Every night we made and refrigerated five 8oz mason jars of coffee enema concentrate. To make the concentrate, we bring five cups of filtered or distilled (preferred) water to a rolling boil. Slowly stir in 1 ¼ cup organic light or medium roast ground enema coffee (¼ cup ground coffee per eight ounces of water).

After the coffee boils, uncovered for 3 minutes, reduce to simmer for 15 minutes covered; cool, strain and pour coffee into the mason jars in equal amounts then top off with filtered or distilled water, cap and refrigerate. (Use one jar of coffee concentrate per enema. Pour coffee into an enema bucket, discarding the residue at the bottom of the jar. Dilute the coffee concentrate with three cups warm distilled or purified water. Repeat for each enema throughout the day.

In the morning I prepared the enema kit which consists of a bucket, tubing and the coffee. Once the bucket is ready, it is time to do the actual enema. Eliminate air bubbles in the tubing by draining some of the coffee through the tubing into the sink until there are no bubbles in the tubing. Use a clamp to stop the coffee flow. Next, place a yoga mat and pillow on the floor and cover the mat with a towel. Then place a disposable pad (Chux) over the towel. Enemas should be administered by lying on the right side, elevating the bucket approximately twelve to eighteen inches above the floor to obtain a slow even flow.

Cleaning the equipment after each use is essential. Use soap like Castile, warm water, and about ¼ cup hydrogen peroxide to clean the bucket. Let the mixture drain through the tubing as well. Rinse the bucket with clean water and let the clean water also drain through the tube for a thorough rinsing. After cleaning the equipment, disinfect the sink with soap and hydrogen peroxide. Also clean the toilet after bowl elimination.

Every other day I replaced one coffee enema with a castor oil coffee enema the first month, then twice a week the remaining two months, then once a month until the end of my two-year program. Castor has many uses. It is filled with vitamin E, proteins, and minerals and has antifungal and antibacterial properties. In this case castor oil is used as a laxative for detoxification. The castor oil coffee enema involves first ingesting two tablespoons castor oil. Yuck! I wash it down with a half cup of sweetened organic coffee and a piece of fruit to cause intestinal stimulation. About an hour later I pour three tablespoons of castor oil in with the coffee enema, and proceed with the enema. (Castor oil treatments are NOT given to patients who have gone or are going through chemotherapy treatments as detoxification can be too rapid and dangerous.)

Even though I have completed my two year therapy, I continue to do a regular coffee enema daily and the castor oil coffee enema once a month. I use them as a personal time to meditate. It is relaxing to me now and is hard for me to believe I was so defiant in the beginning.

During my two-year protocol, we developed a time schedule that proved to work well for us. At first my husband started all the meals and juices until I was able to do them on my own.

Time	Juice	Meals	Five Coffee Breaks
7:00 am		Rise and shine and eat a piece of fruit before doing the morning coffee enema, lovingly referred to as a coffee break, and shower.	
7:45 am		Start breakfast.	
8:00 am	Orange	Breakfast, oatmeal, rye toast with flax oil, fresh juice and supplements with lugol's and potassium follow by a coffee break	Coffee Break
8:30 am		Clean up after breakfast. Wash fruit and vegetables for the day's meals and juices.	
9:00 am	Green	Prepare vegetable juice, referred to as a green juice with potassium. Start "special soup" called Hippocrates Soup for lunch and dinner. It is made fresh each day (leeks, potatoes, tomatoes, onion, celery knob or celery, parsley knob or parsley and vegetable stock)	
9:30 am	Apple/ Carrot	Prepare juice with lugol's and potassium. Take a coffee break.	Coffee Break
10:30 am	Apple/ Carrot	Prepare juice with lugol's and potassium. Take a coffee break.	
11:00 am	Carrot	Prepare juice with liver pills.	
11:30 am	Green	Prepare juice with potassium. Take a coffee break.	Coffee Break
12:00 pm		Prepare lunch with a "special soup" and Gerson approved meal.	
12:30 pm	Apple/ Carrot	Prepare juice with lugol's, potassium and supplements. Eat Gerson approved lunch and "special soup".	
1:00 pm	Green	Prepare juice with potassium. Clean up after lunch.	
3:00 pm	Carrot	Prepare juice with liver pills. Take a coffee break.	Coffee Break
4:00 pm	Green	Prepare juice with potassium.	
5:00 pm	Carrot	Prepare juice with liver pills.	
5:30 pm	Apple/ Carrot	Prepare juice with lugol's and potassium. Start preparing dinner.	
6:00 pm	Apple/ Carrot	Prepare juice with lugol's and supplements. Eat "special soup" with Gerson approved dinner.	
6:30 pm	Apple/ Carrot	Prepare juice. My husband cleans up after dinner while I do my final coffee break.	Coffee Break
7:30 pm		Prepare concentrated coffee for the next day's enemas.	
8:00 pm		Prepare fruit snack plate.	
9:30 pm		Bedtime	

Even though I feel the above juicing schedule is the best for a cancer protocol, it is important to just juice as much as possible and pay attention to what is eaten and change to a new life style in order improve the immune system. Even a blending of fruits and vegetables are better than not juicing at all. It is important that people wanting to heal, at least start juicing and integrating juicing into their daily new lifestyle. Drinking vegetable juices are easier to digest and more nutrition can be obtained than just eating them. I strongly recommend juicing at least two 10 to 12oz vegetable juices a day. These are more important than fruit juices for improving the immune system. Most juicing purists and I may be called one, believe that freshly made juice consumed within twenty minutes of juicing improves the body's ability to use the juice enzymes. However, recent studies have shown that many enzymes are preserved if the juice is kept cold in the refrigerator. Enzyme survival is temperature dependent, and heat can quickly destroy them.

Some cancer patients may not have someone to assist them with daily juicing. New studies have shown that freezing juices can preserve some of the enzymes. Therefore, preparing a batch of juice over the weekend when you may have more time or have someone to help may be an option. Pour the juice in ten ounce mason jars leaving ¼ inch from the top, apply light pressure to seal the lid, and then freeze the jars. Remove what is needed for the next day the night before to thaw in the refrigerator. Please note that these are my suggestions and not recommended by the Gerson Therapy. I am a cancer survivor because of the Gerson Therapy nutrition regimen. However, I feel it is important that those who are unable to do the full therapy should start maximizing their immune system as soon as possible with a "salad drink" of at least five vegetables and only one fruit. A healthy diet should be highly considered for anyone receiving chemotherapy and/or radiation to keep the immune system as healthy as possible.

Periodically throughout the Gerson treatment a person may experience a "healing reaction." It is the body's response, the immune system in particular, causing an increase in the detoxification and healing processes. The body attempts to rid itself of dead and diseased tissue and cells, eliminate toxins of all types, and rebuild healthy cells and tissues.

I had my first "healing reaction" during the first three months of the therapy. I felt like I had the flu and it was difficult to get out of bed. I was depressed. At one point we thought we'd have to get the house fumigated and paint the bathroom from all my toxic releases. WOW! Words cannot describe that. There is a myth that extensive use of enemas could result in dehydration or that the overuse of coffee enemas could result in electrolyte imbalances. I have never had these problems. That is probably because I took supplements and potassium and the fact that there is so much juicing throughout the day while doing the coffee enema detoxification I was never dehydrated.

After the first three months I could definitely feel my body becoming stronger. I no longer felt ill and I was losing weight even while eating three times a day and juicing. Yeah! I started doing my own juicing and preparing our meals. My husband declared that a relief and a victory as he was getting tired of all the preparation. By the sixth month I received approval from my Gerson practitioner to decrease my juice intake to ten per day. The numbers of coffee breaks were lowered to two per day for the rest of my two-year protocol. If I felt I needed an added coffee break, I would do one. At this point, I could add foods like butter, cottage cheese, and yogurt to my diet.

After one year into the Gerson Therapy, I began to return to "normal" life. We had an Airstream trailer and went on a month-long camping road trip. Since I was only drinking ten juices a day and taking two coffee breaks, it felt like I had freedom again. We took our juicer with us and only traveled four hours at a time. When we made camp, I juiced and prepared our meals. After lunch we would decide if we wanted to pack up and continue down the road or stay and visit the local historical sites, go hiking or just relax until it was time to prepare dinner and do more juicing.

After a year and a half I could add eggs and fish back into my diet if I desired, but I chose to wait until after I completed my two-year protocol. I found animal protein to be too hard to digest since my body was no longer used to it. After two years, I did add eggs back to my diet but I could not eat them alone and preferred them mixed with foods. I still don't even like the smell of them raw, which is funny because we live on a farm and raise our own chickens and eggs.

We know exactly what our chickens are fed. Chickens naturally search for food, so we allow them to be free range and forage to supplement their food from nature. We also feed them non-GMO feed or organic feed, when we can get it, and they receive all residual plant material left over from juicing. I do eat fish now, but it is minimal, once or twice a month. I don't have nearly the negative reaction to grilling fish that I do cooking beef, pork, or poultry.

Once our grandkids came to visit and brought hotdogs. Being a good grandma, I cooked them in the kitchen because it was winter. When my husband came into the house, the smell was so overpowering, he actually turned on the ceiling fan and opened all the doors and windows to air out the house. It's striking to remember that we once had no problem cooking meat or eating meat prior the Gerson Therapy. It was a true eye-opener as to how poor meat can be for our bodies. As a result, we no longer allow our grandkids or anyone else for that matter, to cook hotdogs or any meat in the house. Now when they visit and they want meat, it is cooked outside on the gas BBQ. I don't even like the smell of cooked animal meat when we go into a restaurant.

True, the two year Gerson Therapy is an arduous program *in the beginning* and one does need help, just as help is needed when taking chemotherapy. The Gerson Therapy may not be for everyone as everyone's beliefs and circumstances are not the same. But I feel the same is true for chemotherapy and radiation.

I am hoping my story will change the views of many who are "skeptical." I have good results obtained doing the Gerson Therapy. I am well, I am cancer free, I have a healthy heart, I have all my hair, I can be in public without wearing a mask and all my friends and family are free to come and go from our home, sick or not. Cancer changed my life forever and I believe to be for the good! I take great care reading food labels on items my family and I consume as well as what goes on my body.

Chapter Ten

The Importance of Testing and Monitoring Health

THE RESULT OF THE GERSON PROTOCOL has been amazing. I am off all my cholesterol, high blood pressure, and allergy medications. I lost weight and feel healthy. When my weight increases, I pay attention to what I eat, what I am doing and thinking, and I make corrections, and I go back to my desired weight. My husband also lost weight because he did this with me. He is off his acid reflux, high blood pressure and gout medications. He is my biggest supporter and has endured as much as I have doing our lifestyle change. He keeps me on track and stable. He gives me his unconditional love and is my rock.

During the two-year Gerson Therapy, I continued my conventional doctor's visits regularly since there are no blood tests to check for the presence of TNBC. It was important to monitor my breasts through regular mammograms and MRIs of both breasts and brain every three months which eventually changed to every six month. Now I do yearly MRIs. Because I was diligent getting MRIs in particular, a small tumor was detected in my right breast that my routine mammogram did not pick up on January 30, 2013.

My surgeon was concerned that this tumor too could be malignant and recommended it either be biopsied or I have it removed. I elected surgery. Prior to surgery the 5mm nodule of the right breast was localized with ultrasound, a common procedure. My breast was cleansed with antiseptic and was anesthetized. Using a sterile technique, a 5cm localization needle was inserted using real time ultrasound for guidance. A hollow needle was passed through the nodule and an inner wire was deployed into the nodule. The outer needle was removed leaving a wire tip exposed to position the tumor for the surgeon. That day, February 14, 2013, I had surgery, a lumpectomy. The biopsy revealed NO cancer.

A year later almost to the day, February 13, 2014, I had a bilateral digital diagnostic mammogram. No suspicious abnormalities were detected in my right breast; however, the left breast showed a new group of indeterminate calcifications above the postoperative scar. An appointment was immediately arranged with my cancer surgeon. He did a physical exam of both breasts. He observed no lumps and nor could he feel the calcifications around the scar. He then brought the mammogram breast results up on the computer screen and pointed out the location of calcifications. The image showed a mass of little white dots. He gave me two options: more surgery or a biopsy. The biopsy he recommended is called SB-Stereotactic biopsy. My surgeon referred me to a website to learn about the biopsy. I read the description of the procedure and viewed the video. I learned that a stereotactic breast biopsy is a test that uses a special computer to guide a needle to an abnormality seen on mammography. The technique uses a digital imaging device and is less invasive than a surgical biopsy. I felt positive about what I observed, so I chose to have a biopsy.

When I arrived at the hospital on the day of the biopsy, I was brought to a room similar to a mammogram room but with more equipment. I was positioned on my stomach with my right breast placed in a hole so it could be compressed by a mammogram type machine, which could locate the exact position of the calcification.

This device used more compression than I had ever experienced before. It was so excruciating that I nearly passed out from the pain, and I have a high tolerance for pain. When I complained, the nurse said she was sorry but it had to be done this way and to please hold still. The nurse took a picture but I moved. I had to endure a second procedure. This time I held my breath and did not move.

Once the nurse obtained a good picture the doctor came in and examined the images. When he was satisfied and felt he could proceed, he cleansed and anesthetized my left breast while it was under pressure. When I asked why they didn't anesthetize my breast before so much pressure was applied, the nurse said they needed good blood flow for the picture to make sure they marked the correct area for the biopsy. I blurted out, "What blood flow, I am completely compressed!" No more was said.

A breast core biopsy involves a special needle (or probe) that is inserted into the breast to take a small sample of breast tissue from an area of concern which is then sent to a laboratory for testing. Once my breast was numb, the doctor obtained ten cores. Each core required the probe to be turned and twisted to gather the calcification specimens. Thank goodness for being numb. Pictures were taken to confirm that multiple calcifications were within the specimen material to be tested. But not all calcifications were able to be removed from my breast. More pressure was applied to stop the bleeding from the probe procedure. I could feel tears roll down my cheeks. The pain was unbelievable. When the bleeding was successfully stopped, the pressure was lifted and a bandage was place over the incision. My nipple and breast were purple from the pressure, which lasted a couple of hours after the procedure. Needless to say my breast was sore for a few days.

The explanation of the procedure on the website and video did not go into as much detail as I thought it should have and I felt the video did not show the entire procedure. This made me angry and I told my surgeon I made my decision to have the biopsy based on information from the video. Had I really known what the stereotactic procedure actually entailed, I would have opted for surgery. Surgery would have removed all the calcifications so there would be no chance of cancer recurring and I would have had less pain. The best part however, is that the biopsy revealed NO cancer.

I believe that had I not improved my lifestyle these two biopsies could have been cancerous, but who is to really know for sure. I have a full body bone scan yearly now and it continues to reveal that I am cancer free. The same is true for all other MRIs and mammograms I've received these past few years.

After I healed from the stereotactic procedure I wanted to get an opinion from a plastic surgeon regarding breast reconstruction of both breasts. I went to two plastic surgeons. At the first surgeon appointment, I went by myself and told him about my two breast surgeries and the calcification biopsy. I explained that the left breast tumor revealed triple negative breast cancer, the calcification biopsy of the left breast was negative, and the right breast tested negative for cancer. I told him I did not have chemotherapy or radiation. He said triple negative breast cancer was serious and that I should do chemotherapy. He went on to say he could perform the surgery but since I did not have chemotherapy, he was skeptical and that there was no guarantee that cancer would not come back. He felt that reconstruction would be superfluous. I told him that chemotherapy did not guarantee that cancer would not come back either. The entire appointment lasted less than twenty minutes. I left his office deflated and disappointed.

A couple of months later I saw a second plastic surgeon. I told him my situation and he was surprised I was still alive but genuinely happy for me. He showed me what would happen during the reconstructive surgery, which the first surgeon couldn't be bothered to do. He examined by breasts, took measurements, and determined I was a good candidate for the surgery because the scar tissue was minimal. He was very glad I did not do radiation because it damages the blood supply to normal cells and causes problems with breast reconstruction. He said it increased the risk for complications following surgery including infection, delayed healing, tissue breakdown, and fat necrosis. He determined there was no need for breast implants. He went on to say that most of his breast reconstruction patients achieve an acceptable outcome and he felt I would be more than pleased.

The doctor then explained the reconstruction procedure. The left breast would have to be lifted to cover the scaring left from the cancer surgery. The right larger noncancerous breast needed to be reduced and lifted to match the reconstructed cancerous breast and the nipple would need to be relocated.

The excess and stretched skin of the right breast needed to be removed to achieve the best shape and lifted to make it match the left breast. The breast tissues from the inner, outer and upper portions of the right breast would be removed, reducing the three-dimensional size of the breast, lifting the breast tissue, and repositioning the nipple areolar complex. The nipple areola complex would be reduced with a circular incision and a lower vertical midline incision. An infra-mammary fold incision was to be made (the anchor scar). The blood and nerve supply of the nipple areola complex would remain attached to breast tissue to preserves its sensation.

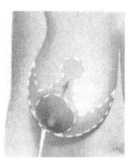 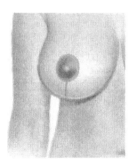

Images were retrieved from http://www.cosmeticsurgeryinreno.com/breast-lift-reno

The outpatient surgery would be performed at a surgery center and would require an overnight stay. General anesthesia, drain tubes to reduce the risk of blood or fluid build-up and to minimize bruising and swelling would be administered. The tubes would be removed between five to seven days after surgery. The breasts would be dressed with gauze and a snug compression dressing for comfort and support. Sutures would be removed seven days after surgery. The recovery time would be four to six weeks.

After much deliberation about what I would have to undergo just to look good, I decided not to have the reconstruction surgery. It took some time for me to come to this conclusion. I thought about all the surgeries I had already gone through during my life time. Doing another one was just too much. My husband also agreed. He said he loved me for who I am and to him what my breasts looked like was minor compared to what I had already gone through. He was grateful I was alive and cancer free and did not hesitate to agree with my decision. So now when I leave the house he makes sure to do what we call a "headlight" check. My right breast nipple angles down and to the right and my left breast nipple is high and to the left. We laugh about this each time I have to adjust my breasts.

Because I had calcifications and still have some in my left breast, I wanted to find out more information about mammograms. My researches lead me to *Mercola.com*. I discovered mammograms use ionizing radiation at a relatively high dose, which can contribute to the mutations that can lead to breast cancer. The body can receive as much radiation from one mammogram as from 1,000 chest X-rays. Mammography also compresses the breasts tightly, which cause pain in some instances, and in other cases the compression may lead to a dangerous spread of cancerous cells, should they exist. Dr. Samuel Epstein, one of the world's top cancer experts, stated: "The premenopausal breast is highly sensitive to radiation, each 1 rad exposure increasing breast cancer risk by about 1 percent, with a cumulative 10 percent increased risk for each breast over a decade's screening." [1]

Further research says that mammograms are NOT really saving lives. In September 2010, the New England Journal of Medicine, one of the most prestigious medical journals, published the first study in years to examine the effectiveness of mammograms.

The study concluded that despite substantial increases in the number of cases of early-stage breast cancer, screening mammography has only marginally reduced the rate at which women present with advanced cancer. The imbalance suggests that there is substantial over-diagnosis, accounting for nearly a third of all newly diagnosed breast cancers, and that screening is having, at best, only a small effect on reducing the rate of death from breast cancer.

Mercola.com further states that these findings are a far cry from what most public health officials would have people believe. The bottom line is that 2,500 women would have to be screened over ten years for a single breast cancer death to be avoided. So according to the research, not only are mammograms unsafe, but they may NOT save women's lives as was commonly thought.

Instead of yearly mammograms I have chosen SonoCiné. SonoCiné is an automated whole breast ultrasound. The computer-guided scanning system uses sound waves to image different tissue structures in women with dense breasts and/or breast implants and women with a family history of breast cancer or a history of biopsy. It is the same technology expectant mothers use to see their unborn babies. It does not require any radiation, breast compression, or injections.

I informed my surgeon of my decision to use SonoCiné instead of mammograms. He said there is nothing wrong with SonoCiné, but he was skeptical of using SonoCiné alone and recommended it be used in addition to a yearly mammogram. SonoCiné, he felt, has yet to be proven as a good stand alone scientific procedure. Here are the words "skeptical" and "scientific" again. We finally came to an agreement that I should have MRIs yearly and six months after the yearly MRI I would do SonoCiné. This way my breasts are checked every six months.

I had my six month checkup as recommended after my calcification biopsy and made an appointment for a SonoCiné screening of both breasts. I was brought into an ultrasound room where my top and bra were removed. A tight fitting mesh camisole was slipped over my head and placed over my breasts and a silicone pad was placed over each nipple under the camisole to flatten the nipples for imaging. I was then asked to lie down on my back on the examination table. A foam pad was placed under the right side of my back for elevation and my right arm was raised above my head. Warm gel was spread over the entire right breast up to the collar bone and the entire armpit area. An imaging wand was pressed firmly and moved slowly in a uniform pattern under the arm, lower lymph nodes, outer breast tissue, clavicle, and inner breast tissue, giving a complete picture of my breast health. This was then repeated on the left breast. The images were formed into a "cine loop" to create a view of my entire breast.

Unlike a mammogram, the examination is painless and only takes about thirty minutes. My results were described as, "No evidence of malignancy to the right breast and postoperative scarring present in the left breast with BIRADS Category of 2-benign findings."

The American College of Radiology (ACR) came up with a standard way to describe imaging findings and results. In this system, the results are sorted into categories numbered 0 through 6. This system is called the Breast Imaging Reporting and Data System (BIRADS). Having a standard way of reporting imaging results lets doctors across the country use the same words and terms, which can help ensure better follow-up of suspicious findings. These categories are used in the official report that goes to the doctor. Different wording is often used in the letters sent to patients. Here's a brief review of the categories.

Category 0: Zero – A zero reading means that a patient needs additional imaging evaluation and/or comparison to prior mammograms or images. This means a possible abnormality may not be clearly seen or defined and more tests are needed, such as the use of spot imaging (applying images to a smaller area), magnified views, special imaging views, or ultrasound. This category sometimes means that the imaging should be compared with older results to see if there have been changes in the area over time.

Category 1: Negative – In Category 1 reading no significant abnormality appears. The breasts are symmetrical with no lumps, distorted structures, or suspicious calcifications. In this category, *negative* means nothing bad was found.

Category 2: Benign (non-cancerous) finding – Category 2 is also a negative image result meaning there's no sign of cancer. However, the reporting doctor chooses to describe a finding known to be benign, such as benign calcifications, lymph nodes in the breast, or calcified fibroadenomas. This label helps others who look at the image to not misinterpret the benign finding as suspicious. This finding is recorded in the image report to help when comparing to future images.

Category 3: Probably benign finding. Follow-up is needed in a short time frame – The findings in Category 3 have a very high chance (greater than 98%) of being benign. The findings are not expected to change over time. But since the area has not been proven benign, it's helpful to see if the area in question changes over time.

Follow-up with repeat imaging is usually done in six months and regularly after that until the finding is known to be stable (usually at least two years). This approach helps avoid unnecessary biopsies, but if the area does change, it still allows for early diagnosis.

Category 4: Suspicious abnormality, Biopsy should be considered – Findings do not definitively look like cancer but could be cancer. The radiologist is concerned enough to recommend a biopsy. The findings in this category can have a wide range of suspicion levels (abnormalities). For this reason, some doctors divide this category further. Not all doctors use subcategories however.

Category 5: Highly suggestive of malignancy, Appropriate action should be taken – The Category 5 findings look like cancer and have a high chance (at least 95%) of being cancer. Biopsy is very strongly recommended.

Category 6: Known biopsy-proven malignancy–Appropriate action should be taken – This category is only used for findings on an image that have already been shown to be cancerous by a previous biopsy. Images may be used in this way to see how well the cancer is responding to treatment.

After understanding BIRADS, I felt more comfortable with my final SonoCiné results of a "Category 2-benign" finding. I have no cancer. It is important also to understand that the $125 cost of the SonoCiné exams are not covered by insurance. The Gerson Therapy cancer program that my husband and I attended at The Longevity Center was less than $7,000 and was not covered by insurance either. The cost of chemotherapy and radiation, had I chosen those treatments, could have been upwards of $300,000 and would have been covered by insurance companies.

It has taken a long time for the medical community at large to see the benefits of a screening process that insurance still does not cover. For me, the added peace of mind that comes from having an additional exam that has proven its ability to find smaller cancers makes the SonoCiné worth the $125 yearly cost. The cost may be higher in some areas but in my area I can receive a discount for the exam during breast cancer awareness month in October.

I had also been thinking about my hormones since my pituitary examinations and blood work reports indicated that my testosterone hormone was low. I decided to make an appointment with my neuroendocrinologist but before I met with him I had another blood test. During my appointment we reviewed my test. My testosterone was still low so I wanted to know the significance of that finding. We discussed hormones at great length. The ovaries produce both testosterone and estrogen. Relatively small quantities of testosterone are released into your bloodstream by the ovaries and adrenal glands as well as estrogen. These sex hormones are involved in the growth, maintenance, and repair of reproductive tissues. They also influence other body tissues and bone mass. At menopause, women experience a decline in testosterone. That decline may be correlated to a reduced libido. Some findings indicate that testosterone replacement therapy may benefit sexual function in certain premenopausal and postmenopausal women. However, because of my TNBC diagnosis he was cautious about hormone replacement recommendations other than testosterone. I asked about bioidentical hormone replacement therapy. The term "bioidentical" means the hor-

81

mones in the product are chemically identical (natural as opposed to synthetic) to those the body produces. Bioidentical hormones have the same exact molecular structure as the hormones produced naturally within the body. The body does not distinguish between supplemental bioidentical hormones and the hormones produced within the body. As a result, bioidentical hormones are able to be naturally metabolized and excreted from the body.

Only bioidentical hormone molecules are indistinguishable from those the body produces and treated the same way by the body. Unnatural synthetic drugs are similar in molecular structure, but are not exactly the same as the bioidentical molecule. Because these synthetic drug molecules are different from natural molecules, the body treats them differently, which can lead to adverse side effects.

My doctor did not have anything against bioidentical hormone replacement therapy but did say insurance wouldn't pay for it because the therapies have not been "scientifically" proven yet and therefore, not approved by the FDA. He said it was up to me and felt that the treatment would probably do no harm.

For decades, physicians prescribed patented non-bioidentical estrogen and progestin drugs, such as Premarin, Provera, and Prempro, to combat the symptoms of menopause. According to the Life Extension Magazine, "Doctors also prescribed non-bioidentical hormones to protect postmenopausal women against osteoporosis and heart disease. Non-bioidentical hormones are not identical in *structure or activity* to the hormones naturally produced within the body. Unfortunately, the logic behind non-bioidentical hormone replacement therapy (HRT) turned out to be fatally flawed. In 2002, the results of a Women's Health Initiative study were released early. This study followed more than 16,000 women and assessed the effects of non-bioidentical hormone replacement therapy (HRT), including estrogen-only therapy and therapy that combined non-bioidentical estrogen and progestin. The findings were shocking: the estrogen/progestin study was terminated early because the non-bioidentical hormone therapy not only failed to protect against heart disease but was shown to increase the risk of heart attack and breast cancer."[2]

Since I had been prescribed Premarin for fifteen years my cancer surgeon suggested that it may have contributed to my cancer but could not say for sure. This was one main reason I did not want any non-bioidentical hormones. However, according to the Food and Drug Administration (FDA) and several medical specialty groups, the hormones marketed as "bioidentical" and "natural" aren't safer than hormones used in traditional synthetic hormone therapy, and there's no "scientific" evidence they're any more effective.

To most people, testosterone is synonymous with masculinity. Although it is classified as one of the androgens, or male hormones, it is vital for *both men and women.* Through ongoing research on women, the medical community is learning that testosterone serves many purposes, ranging from the commonly understood sexual functions to surprising findings that it may help to control blood sugar and may also have an anticoagulant effect. Testosterone also has a role in building muscles and bones that are especially important for women facing age-related disorders such as osteoporosis and cardiovascular disease. Replacing inadequate testosterone with natural testosterone (bioidentical) can help protect the heart, improve mental alertness, make bones stronger, and revive a sagging sex life. Physiological data and clinical outcomes demonstrate that bioidentical hormones are associated with lower risks, including the risk of breast cancer and cardiovascular disease.[3]

For many bioidentical combinations a compounding pharmacy is required, one that specializes in making medications customized for an individual's needs. The products are custom made for the patient, based on testing the unique hormonal needs. I found a doctor specializing in bioidentical hormones and a compounding pharmacy in our area, and made a choice to use bioidentical testosterone cream therapy.

So many times I have been told and continue to be told by my doctors that radiation, which includes mammograms, and drugs are best for treating tumors or hormones and that natural treatment are not the "standard" treatment and therefore unacceptable. They are only unacceptable because they are not approved by the FDA. People must understand that drugs are a big money making business for pharmaceutical companies and are protected by lobbyists. Because of these pharmaceutical companies, bioidentical hormones are not approved by the FDA nor covered by insurance. Alternative programs are not recognized by the FDA so insurance does not cover programs such as The Gerson Therapy or Stanislaw R. Burzynski, M.D., PhD's Burzynski Clinic for brain cancer. Because pharmaceutical companies do not take stock in Samuel S. Epstein, M.D.'s claims on the carcinogenic properties of chlordane pesticides, growth hormones in milk, nitrosamines in bacon, saccharin, beverage preservatives, and other food additives, they are not recognized by the FDA as being harmful. Because pharmaceutical companies do not recognize Dr. Russell Blaylock's discoveries on toxins in food, cookware, and teeth, or that vaccine is a toxic substance that can cause brain damage and are damaging to our immune system, are also not recognized by the FDA as being harmful.

What I have learned healing from cancer is that it is important to monitor my health by proper testing, not using harmful drugs, and keeping my immune system at its optimum. And even though I have had set backs with my health I have learned to take charge of my body because there is no one person who can do that except me.

Chapter Eleven

Overcoming an Unexpected Setback

IN JANUARY OF 2015, I BEGAN TO NOTICE peripheral vision changes and had started to get headaches. I already had my yearly neurosurgeon appointment set up for February, which included an MRI of the brain, so I decided to just wait and go to my scheduled appointment.

My loving husband went with me to my appointment in February. After the MRI, the doctor reviewed the results and asked if I wanted good news or bad news first. "Okay here we go again," I thought. I told him I wanted the good news first. He let me know that I was healthy and my blood tests were good. Whew! The bad news was that I had a macroadenoma (large) tumor, which was putting pressure on the rest of the pituitary gland and could cause problems in nearby structures. The pituitary tumor that was diagnosed in February, 2012 had grown and become so large that it pressed upon my optic nerve and if I did not have brain surgery and have it removed I would go blind. "What? Oh my god!" I immediately felt I was going to throw up and requested a trash can. When my hands started to shake my husband took a hand and put it in his lap. Tears rolled down my cheeks. After I regained my composure I learned I needed to see the neuro-ophthalmologist next to find out how much sight I was losing.

The following week I saw the neuro-ophthalmologist and had a barrage of eye tests. I had a visual field test twice on my left eye to make sure the numbers were correct. Most commonly, visual field test is used for conditions affecting the optic nerve and other forms of neurological disease. The test showed the mean deviation (MD) and the pattern standard deviation (PSD) had changed from the original tests in February 2012.

The mean deviation (MD) is widely used to summarize and interpret various aspects of the visual field. The MD is a representation of the depressed vision for each point when compared with age-matched controls. MD is the average difference from the normal expected value in a particular age group. Typically, an MD of minus 2.00 or less could indicate glaucoma and other eyesight problems.

The pattern standard deviation (PSD) provides information about localized loss—specific area of loss.

In February 2012 my single field of vision for my right eye was in the normal range. The left eye was also in the normal range for my age. In February 2015 my single field of vision for my right eye was outside the normal limits and the left eye was now borderline with MD. The tests were definitive. My eyesight was deteriorating.

I scheduled another appointment to see the neurosurgeon to find out the next step. I wanted to know if the tumor was inside the pituitary as well as surrounding it. I also wanted to know what would happen if I lost the pituitary. The appointment lasted a long time. It appeared the tumor had grown into the pituitary but the doctor was unsure. If I lost the pituitary or if the surgery rendered it nonfunctional, I would have to be on medications for the rest of my life. Thirty years ago people would have died if they lost their pituitary but today medication can correct all the hormonal disorders that arise without a pituitary gland. I learned that it could take up to a year to get the medications under control. The stay in the hospital could be as long as a week in the ICU and an additional three weeks in a regular hospital room if the pituitary was removed.

I asked what would happen if the pituitary sustained no damage. The doctor thought the stay in the hospital could be three days in the ICU and up to four additional days in a regular hospital room. In both scenarios I might need radiation therapy three months after surgery if the entire tumor was unable to be removed. This was not good news.

The Treatment

It turned out I would have a Transsphenoidal surgery on March 11. An ear, nose and throat (ENT) surgeon would perform surgery alongside my neurosurgeon. My doctor said the ENT had done several of these surgeries with him and he was very comfortable with her and her experience. She would make the initial incision inside my mouth under my upper lip and guide him through my nose to the tumor at the base of my brain. After he had removed the tumor, she would close and suture the initial incision.

Transsphenoidal surgery is a type of surgery in which an endoscope and/or surgical instruments are inserted into part of the brain by going through the upper lip, nose and the sphenoid bone (a butterfly-shaped bone at the base of the skull) and then into the sphenoid sinus cavity. Such tumors of the pituitary are within the skull but are outside the brain itself.

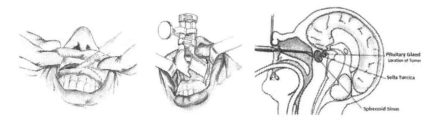

Images retrieved from http://oto.sagepub.com/content/115/1/64/F2. large.jpg

Image retrieved from http://www. health-writings.com/transsphenoidal-pituitary-tumor/

Usually an ENT does not meet the patient until the day of the surgery. However, I wanted to meet her prior to surgery and feel comfortable knowing everyone involved. I met her a week before the surgery. She was very friendly and was glad to meet me. She did a thorough examination and we discussed everything she would be doing during the surgery. She said she had done over 200 of these surgeries 80 with my neurosurgeon and was the only ENT in our area that performed them. She had a good rapport with him and they felt comfortable working with each other. I was relieved and felt comfortable. I was ready for surgery.

Prior to surgery I had a pre-op appointment on March 4th which included blood tests, a chest X-ray, and an EKG. Everything was in order so my surgery was to proceed as planned on March 11th. I checked into a Reno hospital at ten in the morning to complete the necessary paperwork and prepare me for the Transsphenoidal surgery which was scheduled at one in the afternoon. My husband, children, some of my grandchildren, and friends were all at the hospital and were allowed into my pre-op room until I was taken into surgery. I was very afraid and so was my family, but having so many of my immediate family and friends with me gave me comfort.

I don't remember anything after my surgery until the day after. I awoke in the ICU. My neurosurgeon came in and checked my eyes. I could see clearly and had 100 percent of my vision back. I learned the tumor was benign and I would not need radiation.

Despite the good news the recovery was painful. I had dissolvable stitches inside my mouth under my top lip which made it very hard to talk and eat. To stabilize my nose surgical splints were inserted up my nose after surgery which made it very difficult for me to breath and was also very painful. My face was numb and bruised and both my cheeks and upper lip were quite swollen.

I had a tube in my back to drain the overflow of spinal fluid, which is not unusual, but I was having headaches from the pressure of the spinal fluid buildup in my brain. I found the pressure to sometimes be overwhelming. I had an IV for saline solutions and antibiotics, which included a morphine pump equipped with a trigger to press for pain. I only used it when necessary. The remedy for the brain pressure also was to take caffeine to counteract the pain. After the morphine IV pump was removed I took caffeine to relieve the brain pressure. It worked and my headaches diminished somewhat.

Both surgeons thought the surgery would take three hours but it only lasted one and a half hours. My neurosurgeon said the tumor popped out like a big zit after he cut through the bone and he was able to remove the entire tumor without damaging the pituitary. He was amazed. And because he did not remove the pituitary I stayed in ICU for three days and in a regular hospital room for three additional days.

When I returned home, my husband again helped me with the Gerson Therapy to clean my body of all the medications and toxins. I continued to have headaches due to the brain pressure. A week after I was released from the hospital I had a follow up appointment with my ENT to remove my surgical nose splints. This was a huge relief as I could breath freely again. The following week I had a post-op appointment with my neurosurgeon. I asked about the healing process. He said it would take more than a couple of months to heal from the effects of the surgery, including time to heal my mouth, nose, and face from numbness.

I discovered that I also had to be very careful how I ate during my recovery. One day I had to go for a fasting blood test to check my pituitary function as well as test how my liver and kidneys were functioning. I could not eat breakfast and was famished after the tests. We went out to eat and I ordered hot tea with my breakfast. While I drank the tea I could feel the heat on my tongue, but it wasn't until after that I noticed I had burned the roof of my mouth. My mouth and nose were still numb and I had not realized this would be a danger. I had a huge blister as a result. From that day forward I checked to make sure my food was not hot enough to burn my mouth ever again.

I am happy to report that after six months I healed just fine and have my full eyesight back. I am grateful that I had good surgeons and particularly grateful for my neurosurgeon. He was patient with me and listened to my concerns. He did not pressure me to do things I did not want to do; he was kind and compassionate.

Part III

America, Wake-Up

Chapter Twelve

Regulations and Manipulations

TO MAINTAIN A HEALTHY BODY OR keep it healthy after cancer, it is important to understand what may be contributing to the development of cancer and what to do to keep the body from developing cancer. If people are lucky and have not been diagnosed with cancer, then it is important to understand how to keep from developing it as our federal government is not helping or protecting our food supply. This is because we have a problem in our government called the "revolving door".

One thing to remember is that in politics, the "revolving door" is a movement of personnel between roles as legislators and regulators and the industries affected by the legislation and regulation. Michael R. Taylor is a prime example. [1, 2, 3]

With respect to the Food and Drug Administration (FDA), Michael R. Taylor became a staff attorney for the FDA in the 1970s and, over three decades since, has revolved from various departments within the federal government that control our food and King & Spalding Law firm.

Among the law firm's clients was the biotechnology company Monsanto.[3]

During Taylor's employment with the law firm he established and led the firm's food and drug law practice and published an article titled "The De Minimis Interpretation of the Delaney Clause: Legal and Policy Rationale" in the Journal of the American College of Toxicology (now called the International Journal of Toxicology). This publication happened during a debate and litigation over federal agencies' interpretation of the Delaney Clause.

In this country, before food safety became a responsibility of the federal government every state had enacted laws prohibiting the sale of food that contained poisonous substances. Prior to changes of the Delaney Clause which stated, "Provided, that no additive shall be deemed to be safe if it is found to induce cancer when ingested by man or animal, or if it is found, after tests which are appropriate for the evaluation of the safety of food additives, to induce cancer or in man or animal."[4, 5] The Delaney Clause literally prohibited *any* chemical from being added, *in any amount*, to food that was processed, if that agent is carcinogenic.

Later the FDA's risk management approach lowered the levels of carcinogenic agents (pesticides) which changed the interpretation of the Delaney Clause and stated the risk of that carcinogen was "de minimis" (meaning about minimal things) and it could be allowed on the market. [2, 4, 5]

Several years earlier, Congress had amended the federal pesticide statute, the Federal Insecticide, Fungicide, and Rodenticide Act (FIFRA), to require federal registration of any pesticide sold in the United States. FIFRA was the mechanism by which the government—originally FDA and now EPA—assessed the general safety of a pesticide. The Miller Amendments to the Federal Food, Drug and Cosmetic Act (FFDCA) provided the mechanism by which an approved pesticide could lawfully be applied to, and remain on, food sold in interstate commerce.[4, 6, 7]

A further condition of The Food Safety Regulation: Reforming the Delaney Clause was that "the pesticide must have been removed to the extent possible through good processing practices. Congress apparently did not consider the possibility that consumers might ingest larger amounts of some commodities in processed form, which could render any judgment about a pesticide's safety on the raw commodity an unreliable guide to its safety in processed versions." [4] This then means that no consideration of affects caused to the body eating small amounts of food that could build up over a period of time from all the foods that are consumed. One cut will not kill a person but a thousand can.

When Taylor left the law firm again in the 1990s he was given the post of Deputy Commissioner for Policy and later with United States Department of Agriculture (USDA), where he was Administrator of the Food Safety & Inspection Service. During this time he signed a guidance that milk from cows treated with bovine growth hormone (BGH) did not have to be labeled as such and was a co-author of a guidance on genetically modified (GM) plant foods. [1] These two documents meant that the U.S. policy would focus on GM products and techniques, and that only verifiable scientific risks would be tolerated, and that GM products could exist in products. In other words, he was responsible for genetic material in food derived from genetically modified (GM) crops as <u>food additives</u> which were subject to existing food additive regulation. [1, 4, 8]

Our food has been compromised with GM crops and carcinogenic pesticides. This is all because of the change in the Delaney Clause to the De Minimis Interpretation by Mr. Taylor.

GMOs, genetically modified organisms, may be a potential cancer causing agent because of the high use of pesticides. The same chemical companies, Monsanto and Dow to name a few, which manufacture herbicides, have genetically engineered crops such as corn, cotton, and soybeans to *resist* the application of their herbicides. "Technologies like a genetic trait that makes the plants immune to Monsanto's weed killer Roundup make weed control much easier. More than 90 percent of the soybeans grown in the U.S. contain the "Roundup-Ready" trait. Genetic engineering of crops is different from traditional plant breeding because it requires intensive genetic overwriting to allow for genetic changes that cannot occur in nature. Farmers used to save their seeds from their first crop of soybeans from the previous year and use those for second-crop planting after wheat. But that is no longer available as an option because most farmers signed agreements saying they won't do that."[6] This is because in 2013 the Supreme Court upheld patents on Monsanto Biotech seeds: "The seeds of patented plants are patented too, and replanting them violates intellectual property law . . ."[9] Which means farmers could not use the "offspring of plants grown from the company's genetically modified seeds".[6] Monsanto can control our seeds which will control our food. This is not good as some crops are genetically engineered to produce their own pesticides instead of having the pesticides sprayed onto crops or into the soil where they are planted. This type of genetic engineering incorporates a "natural" pesticide from bacteria into the genetic makeup of a crop.[8] And because it is secreted by the plant, it cannot be washed off.

GM crops are promoted as essential for an ever-growing population. However, the findings in the 2009 Failure to Yield Evaluating the Performance of Genetically Engineered Crops, by the Union of Concerned Scientists, reported in detail the overall, or combined, yield effect of GM food. After more than twenty years of research and thirteen years of commercialization in the United States, genetic modifications have done little to increase overall crop yields. Despite this, GM crops account for more than 80 percent of North American crop acreage. Farmers do not choose GM crops. The industry destroys all options.[10]

Globalization of this type is collapsing healthy societies. However, the challenge is to build alternatives before it's too late. As individuals we can save seeds and grow a food garden to restore food sovereignty and build a sustainable society.[10] If everyone had a garden and were able to grow their own food without GM crops, we would have less pesticides and healthier food. It may sound idealistic but in my view, it could happen. There is an old saying "Rome wasn't built in a day."

To better understand what is happening to our food, I need to impart a personal story of what we have observed in our country during the months of July and August 2014. My husband and I took a six week camping vacation, touring some of the northern and Midwestern states, which included parts of Idaho, Montana, both the Dakotas, Minnesota, Washington, and Wyoming along the main highways—2, 5, I-80, I-15, I-25, and I-90.

Food on these routes was okay but not as healthy as we were used to and it was hard to find organic food. We reached my sister's home in Minnesota and were happy to obtain organic food from stores and local farmers markets that used no pesticides or non-GMO products. My juicing could commence regularly again.

After a few weeks we departed Minnesota to visit an elderly aunt and cousin who now own our family's farm in North Dakota. We saw the harvesting of canola, soybean, and wheat. While we were overlooking the wheat, my cousin groaned, lamenting that someone had been driving through their wheat field again and pointed at the tracks.

On the way back to the farm house I noticed more tracks in another wheat field and I pointed them out. My cousin said that was not their property and those tracks were deliberate. She said their neighbors spray "Roundup" (produced by Monsanto) on their wheat to kill it (this allows for rapid dry down) so they can harvest earlier. My husband and I glanced sideways at each other, appalled. She must have seen our expressions as she quickly reassured us that they do not use "Roundup" for that purpose and allowed nature to tell them when it was time to harvest and hoped their crops would not be affected by that type of treatment.

We said our goodbyes and departed for home via highway 5 and 2, the northern route. These routes are where we discovered how poor the quality of food was and how poorly this part of our country eats. Large grocery stores are few and far between, literally. We found no organic food and were given strange looks when we inquired about an organic section. Trying to stay on a healthy vegetarian organic diet was proving to be very difficult.

The restaurants generally served copious types of hamburgers, greasy pan-fried or deep fried meats and fish with fried, boiled, baked or mashed potatoes, overcooked (usually canned) peas, carrots, or corn. The salads were mainly iceberg lettuce with some tomato and served with canned dressing. These types of foods generally have large amounts of salt and saturated fat.

North Dakota and Montana primarily grow wheat, soybeans, and corn. Because of our new found knowledge from my cousin about Roundup, we began to notice the fields. Of the crop fields we noticed approximately 50 percent had tracks running through them. We also observed how they were beginning to turn dark gray in color and die. We had no idea that crop dusting was still being used and witnessed several small aircraft spraying, what could be assumed were chemicals or pesticides, over crops of soybean and corn.

People, we are not only eating unhealthy GMO food because of the political influences, but we are eating contaminated food that we witnessed firsthand! Washing crops is not going to rid the pesticides out of the soybean and corn. Wheat and corn are harvested to be processed and used in all sorts of the food we eat, including flours and cereals we feed our children.

America, Wake Up!

Chapter Thirteen

Produce and Pesticides

WE KNOW THAT PESTICIDES ARE known carcinogens and pesticide residue on some fruits and vegetables are a concern to me. The risk from pesticides on conventionally grown produce can vary from very low to very high, and it depends on the type of produce and the country where it's grown. For these reasons, I shop for organically or locally grown fruits and vegetables and I always ask the local farmers if they use pesticides or GMO products. Being diagnosed with cancer has made me more aware of what goes in and on my body. Reading labels and asking questions about my products will help me be healthier and have less chance of cancer recurrence. Pesticides are making us ill and we must pay attention! Being aware will help our children and our environment.

Mary Ellen Kustin, a senior policy analyst with Environmental Working Group (EWG) said "We are truly disappointed in the USDA for putting the interests of chemical companies before the health of our children and the environment. Instead of putting the brakes on the chemical treadmill, the government is on the fast track to approve more toxic weed killers. The USDA's decision to approve new varieties of genetically engineered corn and soybean seeds brings us one step closer to widespread use of a new toxic weed killer that would threaten children's health and the environment." [1]

The USDA's decision allows chemical manufacturer Dow Agro Sciences to sell 2,4-D and glyphosate-tolerant corn and soybean seeds with its new weed killer, known as Enlist Duo. This pesticide is now awaiting approval from the U.S. Environmental Protection Agency to sell Enlist Duo, a toxic combination of 2,4-D and glyphosate. The company wants to market its new product to farmers who are inundated with the hardy weeds that have evolved to tolerate glyphosate, which is the active ingredient in Monsanto's popular weed killer, "Roundup".[1] Human exposure to 2,4-D has been linked to non-Hodgkin lymphoma, Parkinson's disease and thyroid problems. EWG also contends that the new herbicide could spur the evolution of new "superweeds" resistant to both 2,4-D and glyphosate.

If the EPA approves Enlist Duo, nationwide use of 2,4-D could more than triple by 2020. Communities near sprayed crop fields could have up to eight times more of the chemical exposure than they do today. More than 480 elementary schools nationwide are within 200 feet of corn and soybean fields that could be blanketed by the new weed killer. According to Kustin, "Tens of thousands of young children would be exposed to more intense concentrations of a toxic defoliant that is linked to cancer than is the case today. The EPA must go back and do a thorough assessment of the serious risks associated with 2,4-D. Once that's done, it will be hard not to conclude that approving Enlist Duo is not the right decision for our children and the environment." [1]

According to a thirty page Consumer Report from May 2015, there is core evidence that the way food is produced has an impact on public health. A farmer today finds labor intensive hand weeding methods to be old-fashioned and costs too much money. Since the industrial revolution in the mid 1800s, chemical-based pesticides have been widely used growing crops. Farmers use nearly 700 million pounds of pesticides every year. The pesticide use not only affects the consumers who eat the treated crops but also harms the farm workers, rural residents, and wild-life.

The negative effects of pesticides can remain in the soil long after the pests have died from the pesticides used to kill them. We are still living with the consequences of the pesticides that were used generations ago such as DDT, which has been proven to be carcinogenic and causes increased tumor production. DDT was banned more than forty years ago, but it can still be found in foods today, such as dairy, potatoes, and meat. By eating these foods, we are still at major risk of exposure. According to Environmental Health News, reports show that birds are still dying from DDT in towns where the pesticide was manufactured more than 50 years ago. "The birds apparently have been poisoned by eating worms living in contaminated soil near the old chemical plant."[2]

The American Academy of Pediatrics (AAP) points out that "Children encounter pesticides daily in air, food, dust, and soil and on surfaces through home and public lawn or garden application, household insecticide use, application to pets, and agricultural product residues. For many children, diet may be the most influential source, as illustrated by an intervention study that placed children on an organic diet (produced without pesticide) and observed drastic and immediate decrease in urinary excretion of pesticide metabolites."[3] Studies have shown that children exposed to pesticides have a greater risk of "preterm birth, low birth weight, congenital anomalies, pediatric cancers, neurobehavioral and cognitive deficits, asthma, and adverse neurodevelopment. Multiple case-control studies and evidence reviews indicate exposure to insecticides increase the risk of brain tumors and acute lymphocytic leukemia."[4]

It is difficult to get laws that prevent pesticide use to change because much of the scientific evidence and data that the Environmental Protection Agency (EPA) reviews and relies upon in making its decisions during its risk assessment of products are provided by the companies seeking pesticide registration. And, the safety testing by BioMed Research International, assumes that higher doses are more harmful than lower doses of an individual pesticide. Chemical mixtures are largely untested and their effects are unknown because testing is generally done on individual pesticides rather than on mixtures. [5]

Children exposed to pesticides known as organophosphates (a group of chemicals that have many household and commercial uses, but are commonly used as insecticides and are responsible for a number of poisonings) could have a higher risk of attention-deficit/hyperactivity disorder (ADHD), according to a U.S. study that urges parents to always wash produce thoroughly. "Researchers tracked the pesticides' break-down products in children's urine and found those with high levels were almost twice as likely to develop ADHD as those with undetectable levels." [5] Children with higher pesticide exposure also have higher rates of IQ deficits and behavioral problems.

On June 1, 2010, CNN posted a study from an Environmental Working Group (EWG) report that analyzed the presence of pesticides on produce. The group, a nonprofit focused on public health, scoured nearly 100,000 produce pesticide reports from the U.S. Department of Agriculture and the U.S. Food and Drug Administration to determine what fruits and vegetable have the highest and lowest amounts of chemi-cal residue. Most alarming are the fruits and vegetables dubbed the "Dirty Dozen," which contain 47 to 67 pesticides per serving. For exam-ple, non-organic celery may contain up to 67 pesticides. These twelve foods are believed to be most susceptible because they have soft skin that tends to absorb more pesticides.

The Dirty Dozen include: celery, peaches, strawberries, apples, domestic blueberries, nectarines, sweet bell peppers, spinach, cherries, potatoes, imported grapes and lettuce.

Not all non-organic fruits and vegetables have a high pesticide level. The group found a number of non-organic fruits and vegetables dubbed the "Clean 15" that contained little to no pesticides.

The Clean 15 include: onions, avocados, sweet corn, pineapples, mango, sweet peas, asparagus, kiwi fruit, cabbage, eggplant, cantaloupe, watermelon, grapefruit, sweet potatoes, and sweet onions. [6]

EWG's Amy Rosenthal emphasizes the importance of consumer awareness when it comes to buying produce: "It is critical people know what they are consuming. The list is based on pesticide tests conducted after the produce was washed with USDA high-power pressure water system. The numbers reflect the closest thing to what consumers are buying at the store."[6] The group suggests limiting consumption of pesticides by purchasing organic varieties of the twelve fruits and vegetables on the "Dirty Dozen" list. "You can reduce your exposure to pesticides by up to 80 percent by buying the organic version of the Dirty Dozen,"[6] Rosenthal said.

Americans now eat four times as many fresh strawberries as they did in the 1970s and it is sad to say that strawberries, if not organic, are the worst fruit of all to eat. "U.S. Department of Agriculture (USDA) found that a single sample of strawberries contained 13 different pesticides. Growers of nonorganic strawberries in California—where nearly 90% of the nation's strawberries are produced—continue to pump hazardous substances into fields." [7] This is because in 2002, Paul Helliker of the California Department of Pesticide Regulation, allowed some growers to ignore the restrictions for a pesticide commonly used on strawberries called 1,3-Dichloropropene (1,3-D), a gas injected into the soil before planting crops such as strawberries and almonds. California believed 1,3-D caused cancer. However, because of a loophole growers in communities across the state legally can use 1,3-D at levels that state scientists have said are unacceptable that was only to be temporary. Helliker gave Dow (the company that manufactures 1,3-D) and growers two years to come up with a plan to follow his department's rules or to create new ones. It took Dow less than a year to hand in its proposal. The company's plan didn't close the loophole but it greatly expanded it. Dow asked that the director allow growers across the state to use twice as much 1,3-D in a year as the rules permitted. And the company wanted it to happen quickly. Two Dow officials, Bryan Stuart and Bruce Houtman, closed their proposal by saying that "implementation will begin immediately upon receipt of approval." [8] "Six days later, Helliker signed off on the heart of Dow's plan, which dismantled the strict oversight designed seven years earlier to protect Californians from cancer, opening the door to twelve years of nearly unfettered 1,3-D access as its use spread to populated areas near schools, homes and businesses." [8]

Another pesticide found in conventionally grown fruits and vegetables is organophosphorous pesticide also known as chlorpyrifos. It is also found in some of our drinking water. Chlorpyrifos is known for its damaging effects on the human nervous system which blocks an enzyme (called acytyl cholinesterase) that our brains need to control nerve impulses. These neurological impulses especially affect children because their nervous systems are still developing. This pesticide is prone to drift or become airborne especially when outdoor temperatures are high. Once in gas form, the neurotoxin can migrate to nearby homes and schools, putting residents and their children at risk. [9]

Chlorpyrifos has been banned in the home (aerosol pest control) because of the dangers to children. However, chlorpyrifos is still heavily used on fruit, nut orchards, soybeans, and corn, with an estimated five million pounds applied in the U.S. annually. This means that people continue to be exposed by contaminated foods and drinking water from pesticides drifting from farmlands and into neighboring areas. For this reason in "September 2014 a coalition of environmental health groups, including Pesticide Action Network North America (PANNA), filed a renewed petition for a writ of mandamus seeking an order from the Ninth Circuit Court requiring the EPA to respond to a 2007 petition to ban uses of chlorpyrifos." [10]

According to the Ninth Circuit Court petition, the "EPA has initiated several processes to assess the health risks posed by chlorpyrifos as presented in the 2007 petition and has released some partial responses that address discrete contentions. The EPA has agreed to establish no-spray stream buffer zones in California, Oregon, and Washington to protect salmon from pesticides, including chlorpyrifos. However, it has yet to issue a final and reviewable decision on the request to ban chlorpyrifos, leaving PANNA in legal limbo and this dangerous pesticide in widespread use. Over the past several years, the EPA has made commitments to PANNA and the courts to resolve the 2007 petition and decide whether to ban chlorpyrifos by various deadlines. Without fail, the EPA has violated these commitments and it is unclear as to when this will be resolved. The counsel information for the EPA was not available and said it does not comment on pending litigation."[11]

A Harvard University study of pesticides in males who consumed fruits and vegetables with relatively large amounts of pesticide residue found that men's sperm counts may be affected. "Consumption of fruits and vegetables with high levels of pesticide residues was associated with a lower total sperm count and a lower percentage of morphologically normal sperm among men presenting to a fertility clinic."[12] Furthermore, the study by the researchers at the Harvard T.H. Chan School of Public Health, described pesticides in fruits and vegetables as a link to reproductive problems. Because of the study's design however, the researchers could not determine whether the pesticide residue *caused* the problems they found in the sperm of 155 men who provided samples at a fertility clinic. But the results were clear enough: "Low-to-moderate pesticide residue fruit and vegetable intake was associated with a higher percentage of morphologically normal sperm."[12]

The March 30, 2015 Washington Post also ran an article on men's fertility and pesticides stating that "The researchers used U.S. Department of Agriculture data to classify the levels of pesticide residue in 35 fruits and vegetables between 2006 and 2012. They asked 155 men how much of each they ate (they averaged 0.9 daily servings of high-pesticide produce and 2.3 servings of low-to moderate-pesticide fruits and vegetables), then checked their semen samples for a variety of problems. When they ruled out smoking, obesity, age, physical activity and other factors, they found that men who consumed the largest amounts of high-residue fruits and vegetables had 49 percent lower sperm counts, 32 percent fewer normal-appearing sperm and a 29 percent lower ejaculate volume than men who ate the smallest amounts of those fruits and vegetables."[13]

Many studies have been performed on the adverse effects of pesticides and have proven that pesticides are designed to be toxic to living organisms. Rural residents have been exposed to 2,4-D and other chlorophenoxy herbicides and are listed as 2B carcinogens or, "possibly carcinogenic to humans." Chlorophenoxy compounds are sometimes mixed into commercial fertilizers to control growth of broadleaf weeds. Studies show an association between cancer mortality and living near farm fields treated with the herbicide 2,4-D. These compounds are irritating to skin and mucous membranes and cause vomiting, diarrhea, headache, confusion, bizarre or aggressive behavior, peculiar odor on breath, metabolic acidosis, renal failure, and tachycardia (an abnormally rapid heart rate). Atrazine, another herbicide, is used to prevent broadleaf weeds from starting to grow or to kill them as they grow in crops such as maize (corn), excluding sweet corn, and sugarcane and on turf, such as golf courses and residential lawns and has been found in water supplies. Atrazine is suspected to interrupt the endocrine development, which may affect reproductive health and children's sexual development. "Although the U.S. Environmental Protection Agency (EPA) approved its continued use in October 2003, that same month the European Union (EU) announced a ban of atrazine because of ubiquitous and unpreventable water contamination."[14]

Farmers and farm workers also face high risk of exposure to pesticides given their proximity to the chemicals. High pesticide exposure among farmers has been linked to prostate and ovarian cancer, lung cancer, stomach cancer, hypothyroidism, changes in memory and attention, and increased respiratory disease. Additionally, 10,000 to 20,000 pesticide poisonings occur each year among farmers and farm workers. Mild Poisoning or early symptoms of acute poisoning may include: headache, fatigue, weakness, dizziness, restlessness, nervousness, perspiration, nausea, diarrhea, loss of appetite, loss of weight, thirst, moodiness, soreness in joints, skin irritation, eye irritation, irritation of the nose and throat.

With all the health problems we are facing in America with the use of pesticides in conventional farming, it is time for everyone to take food more seriously. I believe we all should think and eat organic. The March 2015 Consumer Reports issue "From Crop to Table" states that organic farmers are held to the highest standards in food production.

Federal law prohibits the use of almost all synthetic pesticides, insecticides and herbicides on organic farms as well as to maintain buffer zones to prevent inadvertent contamination by synthetic farm chemicals from adjacent conventional fields. But what are the differences between pesticides, insecticides and herbicides?

Pesticides are chemicals that may be used to kill fungus, bacteria, insects, plant diseases, snails, slugs, or weeds. These chemicals can work by ingestion or by touch and death may occur immediately or over a long period of time. All organophosphate pesticides and synthetic soil fumigants (fumigation is a method of pest control that completely fills an area with gaseous pesticides—or fumigants—to suffocate or poison the pests within) are prohibited on organic farms.

Insecticides are a type of pesticide that is used to specifically target and kill insects. Some insecticides include snail bait, ant killer, and wasp killer. All neonicotinoids (insecticide resembling nicotine) are prohibited on organic farms.

Herbicides are used to kill undesirable plants or "weeds". Some herbicides will kill all the plants they touch, while others are designed to target one species. There are currently no synthetic herbicides approved for use on organic food crops. The herbicide glyphosate is prohibited on organic farms. The herbicide atrazine is prohibited on organic farms.

In order for farmers to say their crops are organic the food must be "certified" organic by the USDA guidelines. For certification, organic farmers complete an annual submission of an organic system plan (a detailed description of practices and procedures to be performed and maintained, management practices and physical barriers established to prevent commingling of organic and nonorganic products and changes that may occur in the upcoming year) and the farm fields and processing facilities must be inspected. The inspectors verify that organic practices such as long-term soil management, buffering between organic farms and neighboring conventional farms, and recordkeeping are being followed. The processing inspector reviews the facility's cleaning and pest control methods, ingredient transportation and storage, and recordkeeping and audit control. Organic foods are minimally processed to maintain the integrity of food without artificial ingredients or preservatives and there must not be any use of synthetic agrochemicals, irradiation and genetically engineered foods or ingredients.[15] Since 2002, the USDA National Organic Program (www.ams.usda.gov/nop) "certifies" the farm as an organic agency and also oversees the regulatory process.

There has been no definitive study that organic food is more *nutritious* than conventional food. However, a 2002 report (Baker, B.P., C.M. Benbrook, E. Groth III, and K.L. Benbrook.2002) indicates that organic food is far less likely to contain pesticide residues than conventional food (13% of organic produce samples vs. 71% of conventional produce samples contained a pesticide residue, when long-banned persistent pesticides were excluded).[16]

There are many differences between organic and conventional farming and the arguments whether or not conventional farming methods are safe for someone's health is the most concerning. This is because of the pesticides and GMO's used in the conventional farming practices. Many people are concerned that those growing practices promote unsafe chemical use. The conclusion is obvious to me. Americans need to eat more fruits and vegetables, promote good eating habits by making choices based on health, and moreover avoid harmful pesticides, "buy organic".

America, Wake Up!

Chapter Fourteen

Not Eating Meat and Why

ABOUT 25 YEARS BEFORE I WAS diagnosed with cancer, I loved to eat a good steak or hamburger. At some point I began to notice that every time I ate red meat I became ill the next day. It was like I had a hangover. I was literally sick to my stomach and had diarrhea. With that awareness, I gave up eating any type of red meat and noticed my overall health felt better. A few years later, I had a problem digesting pork, the other white meat. I noticed that most of the time when I ate, pork chops, ham, sausage or bacon I became ill with, nausea and diarrhea. One time in particular after eating bacon I got extremely ill. I had a tremendous pain in my stomach, chest and mid back. My husband brought me to emergency and shortly after, my gallbladder was removed. My doctor said I was probably consuming too much fatty or greasy meat. I gave up pork.

Studies have shown that going meatless once a week may reduce your risk of chronic preventable conditions like cancer, cardiovascular disease, diabetes and obesity. Until 2009, the argument to reduce the consumption of meat was dietary. It was to cut back on saturated fat, lower cholesterol, and reduce the risk of heart disease and other chronic illnesses. But meat eaters have many additional factors to consider as to whether the conventional health advice is still sound.

The public health goals of regulation were to assure that drugs were safe and effective in animals and that any residues in food derived from such animals could be safely consumed by humans.[1] There has been more concern about industrial meat because of the environmental impact, inhumane animal conditions, and because too many antibiotics are fed to animals that are consumed for food.[2]

The three most consumed types of animal protein in this country are beef, chicken, and pork. They are produced on enormous industrial scale farms sometimes referred to as animal feeding operations (AFOs). These agricultural enterprises raise animals in confined situations. AFOs congregate animals, feed, manure and urine, dead animals, and production operations on a small land area. Feed is brought to the animals rather than the animals grazing or otherwise seeking feed in pastures, fields, or on rangeland. There are approximately 450,000 of these AFOs in the United States which accounts for 97 percent of U.S. beef cattle that are on AFO.[2, 3, 4]

Concentrated Animal Feeding Operations (CAFOs) is another term for a large concentrated AFO. A CAFO is an AFO with more than 1000 animal units (an animal unit is defined as an animal equivalent of 1000 pounds live weight and equates to 1000 head of beef cattle, 700 dairy cows (heavier than beef cattle), 2500 swine weighing more than 55 lbs each, 125,000 broiler chickens, or 82,000 laying hens or pullets) confined on site for more than 45 days during the year.[2, 3, 4]

On these factory farms, animals eat commodity GM crops of primarily corn and soybeans which are subsidized by tax-payers via the Farm Bill.[2] So 149 million acres in the US produces animal feed from GM crops designed to resist weed killers such as Roundup. In addition, anabolic steroids are typically used in combinations. Measurable levels of growth-promoting hormones are found at slaughter in the muscle, fat, liver, kidneys and other organ meats, which according to the Food and

Drug Administration are "acceptable daily intakes" (ADIs) for these animal drugs.[5]

Beef cattle are given anabolic steroids as well as estrogen, androgen and progestin, commonly called bovine growth hormones (BGH), developed by Monsanto,[1,5,6] to make them put on weight more quickly. "Although the European Union banned the use of these hormones in 1988, they are still commonplace in the United States." [5] Every beef eating American, for more than 50 years, has been exposed to steroids and growth hormones. Pigs, too, are fed growth hormones. However, the use of growth hormones in poultry has been illegal in the United States since the 1950s. [2,5,6]

Many large scale dairy farms also give their cows growth hormones and according to Organic Consumers: "The congressional General Accounting Office has warned of the potential human health hazards from the consumption of milk or flesh (about 40% of the beef used to make hamburgers come from "old" dairy cows) derived from BGH-treated cows. The Consumer's Union went on to state that the FDA should not have even approved it. BGH "treatment" causes significantly increased levels of another growth hormone called IGF-1 in the milk, according to a 1990 study sponsored by Monsanto and published in Science." [6]

Despite nationwide protests by consumer groups, in 1994 Monsanto and the FDA forced onto the US market the world's first genetically engineered (GE) animal drug, recombinant Bovine Growth Hormone (rBGH, sometimes known as rBST). The FDA's approval was based solely on one study administered by Monsanto. BGH is a powerful GE drug produced by Monsanto which, injected into dairy cows, forces them to produce 15%-25% more milk (to make more money), in the process seriously damaging their health and reproductive capacity.[6] Regardless of warnings from scientists, such as Dr. Michael Hansen from the Consumers Union and Dr. Samuel Epstein from the Cancer Prevention Coalition, that milk or beef from rBGH injected cows contains substantially higher amounts of a potent colon and breast cancer tumor promoter called IGF-

1, and despite evidence that rBGH milk or meat contains higher levels of pus, bacteria, and antibiotics, the FDA gave the hormone its seal of approval, with no real pre-market safety testing required.[3,6] Since rBGH was approved, approximately 40,000 small and medium-sized US dairy farmers, 1/3 of the total in the country, have gone out of business because they cannot compete with the low milk prices produced by the industrial-sized dairies, most of whom are injecting their cows with this cruel and dangerous drug.[6,9] According to the Center for Food Safety almost 50 percent of milk in the US has rBGH which also effects cheese, yogurt and ice-cream.

Antibiotics and pollutants are another problem the US faces from livestock farming. About 80 percent of all antibiotics sold in the U.S. are administered to livestock, a figure acknowledged by the U.S. Food and Drug Administration (FDA) in 2010 and 2011.[3, 7, 8, 9]

However, the information gathered does not include essential details, such as the species of animal receiving the drugs so it is hard to say for sure how much goes to which animal. But 80 percent, to me, is a high number to be given to livestock which the US consumes.

Civil Eats published an article, *Antibiotics Used in Livestock*, in September, 2013 posed a question that if antibiotics kill microorganisms in animals' guts what would be the effects on humans consuming meat from animals injected with antibiotics. In August, 2013, a paper published in *Nature*, "identifies a correlation between diversity of gut microflora and human obesity. A nine-year study, led by Dr. S. Dusko Ehrlich of France's National Institute for Agricultural Research, compared microbiotas–the 100-trillion-member microbial ecosystems that populate the body–of slim and obese people.[10]

The team found obese people have lower microbial diversity in their bellies. This is consistent with earlier research in mice, as well as a paper published last year in Journal of Obesity that found a strong correlation between young children's exposure to antibiotics and later obesity. However, more significantly, the team behind the *Nature* study found a correlation between low microbial diversity and heart disease, diabetes and cancer, regardless of weight."[10]

Air pollution from agriculture is a reasonably new phenomenon. When the Clean Air Act (CAA) was drafted in 1970, legislators excluded agriculture, since at that time farms could hardly be considered serious sources of air pollution. The traditional "family" farm, the dominant agricultural model when the CAA emerged, is relatively small in scale and light on the land, and not a serious pollution threat. Farming, however, is not what it once was. The United States still has large numbers of family farmers; however this group is quickly diminishing. Industrial agriculture is an entirely new breed of farming and is replacing the family farm. According to the National Water Quality Inventory 2004 report, the top reported sources of impairment in assessed rivers and streams are from the Agricultural activities, such as crop production, grazing, and animal feeding operations are the number one sources of pollutants.[3,4,11]

Notwithstanding the numerous problems associated with AFOs, or "factory-style farms," they have displaced the family farms, have caused the destruction of rural communities, animal welfare concerns, and human health problems.[3] AFO commodities are killing our food source and us.

An Agricultural Health Study to evaluate cancer risk associated with raising animals as commodities revealed that raising poultry was associated with an increased risk of colon cancer with further increased risk of non-Hodgkin lymphoma. Raising sheep was associated with a significantly increased risk of multiple myeloma and raising livestock was a lung cancer risk.[12]

In October, 2015 the World Health Organization has deemed that processed meats—such as bacon, sausages and hot dogs—can cause cancer. Although "eating meat has known health benefits, it also points out that the cancer risk increases with the amount of meat consumed."[13]

Because the risks and the benefits vary by product—meat is different from produce. There are problems with E. coli in organically grown and conventionally grown produce and with salmonella in organically raised and conventionally raised chicken and other meats. However, there are more concerns of high pesticide residue in conventionally grown produce and antibiotics and hormones in milk and meat products conventionally raised. Organic milk or meats do not contain antibiotics or hormones.

The consumption of beef, pork, and lamb should be limited to once every two weeks. All meat including poultry that is consumed should be organic grass fed, flax fed or wild game. If not, eat meat at your own risk.

America, Wake Up!

Part IV

Changes, Knowledge, Diets and Other
Maintenance

Chapter Fifteen

Change in Attitude

IN ORDER TO COMPLETELY HEAL, I NOT only had to change my lifestyle, I had to change my attitude. When I was first diagnosed with breast cancer, I worried about my family and had an overwhelming feeling of fear. How will they get along without me? What about my husband? What was he going to do? How and what will I tell my friends? How was I going to tell my boss? I had been employed at a job I loved for seventeen years as a controller/secretary-treasurer. I had been with them through good times and the bad economic times. How could I leave them? I liked the hundreds of people who worked there. I finally came to the conclusion that I was not irreplaceable and held to the idea that they would find someone who might be better than me to bring them forward. It was a difficult time and hard to accept but I retired and began my healing process inside and out.

Moving from fear to gratitude

The biggest thing for me in changing my attitude was getting rid of the fear. Fear is **f**alse **e**vidence **a**ppearing **r**eal. Something that appears to be real is really the fear of the future, but the future is not happening now. There is no need to have fear because I can only control the here and now. I realized that if I was going to succeed in beating cancer, I had to understand that cancer was not a death sentence. Everyone will die sooner or later. I didn't need to learn how to fight death. I had to learn how to fight cancer, how to make my body strong, and feed the life in me and live!

Changing the way I eat, my thoughts, my morale, and exercise was not a change that came fast or easily. It took time! It takes work to be healthy. Hard work!

I also had to change my attitude about exercise. I used to walk four miles every day when I was in my thirties and forties and I have no idea why I stopped. I am in my sixties now and I started again. I suggest that everyone needs to exercise but should consult their doctor to see what exercise is appropriate for them. Even if it is just a short walk or a little yoga (try Yoga for Beginners on DVD, which can be purchased from www.raviana.com), something is better than nothing. My husband and I hike or walk for exercise every day and we meditate. Did you know that meditating just five minutes throughout the day can relieve stress and will allow you to become more productive? Even if at work, take one or two five minute breaks to meditate. Just sit straight, close your eyes and concentrate on breathing. There should be no interruptions so leave the cell phone behind. Go outside or to the bathroom if necessary to get away from distractions. If the mind wanders, and it will, go back and concentrate on breathing. Meditation is easy once you practice it. Meditation relieves stress and helps me change my attitude and be more positive and grateful. Attitude is gratitude and gratitude is attitude. Changing my attitude about my eating habits was the hardest, but once I made that change, the rest was easy.

Accepting others for who they are

When I passed the one year mark of my cancer diagnoses, I realized I had really made the right choice. I was still alive! My life had changed and I had changed. I saw life positively rather than negatively. My attitude toward people changed. I had learned I can't change the way people are, how they look, what they do or don't do. I now accept people more for *who* they are. I have become an "allower," meaning I allow people to be themselves and accept that people have the right to be or do whatever they want. I am powerless to change their thoughts. I can share information but it is up to them to do what they want to do. However, I learned I can help when I can, if I am allowed.

I am more grateful for everything and give thanks daily. I am calmer, happier, and not as frantic for what the future may bring. It is today, it is now. I have more respect for my children and allow them to be who they are. I love them more. The same is true for the rest of my family and friends. My husband and I celebrate the anniversary of my diagnosis as my first day of life. I give thanks for *life* every day.

If I see someone alongside a street holding a sign asking for food or money, I don't feel a negative thought as I once did. I think a good thought for that person and know he or she will find what he or she needs. One day I noticed a man standing on the street corner near the grocery store where I shop. He held a sign that said, "I need money for food and gas. I am stranded." I paid no further mind to him. I went into the store and completed my shopping, leaving with a container of organic vegetable soup and a sourdough roll to eat on my way home. I got into my car and proceeded out of the parking lot. As I did I took note of the man again. He was still there. At that moment, I had an overwhelming feeling that he really was hungry. So I stopped and gave him my lunch. The look on his face was one of complete gratitude and that made me feel gratitude as well.

If I see something I like in a person, I feel more free to express that to them. One day a woman walked by me on my way into a store and I noticed the lovely lace blouse she was wearing. I commented to her how pretty I thought it was. She looked at me, smiled, and said she liked it too and how it reminded her of her 1960 hippy days. She stayed next to me and as we walked into the store together she relayed that memories were all she had now because her body was giving out but that day was a good day as she had energy and could go shopping. For some reason I didn't sympathize. Instead I congratulated her for having a good day and said "Aren't you grateful?" She took her cart, started into the store, turned to me and said "Yes, thank you." That was another opportunity to feel gratitude.

Resisting change

People say the darnedest things when they don't want to change: "I can't do what you are doing" or "man it sure must be hard to give up meat and bread." I even had one person tell me, "You gave up alcohol? Pity!" I have had people say that organic food is too expensive or that they can't afford to be an organic vegetarian or that it is just too expensive to buy a juicer and too hard do all that juicing or that juicing is too time consuming. Now to me, those are just excuses. My answer is, "Is it expensive to pay for a doctor's visit or a trip to the emergency room? Is it too expensive to pay for medication every week or every month? How easy is it to take time out of *your* day to attend a doctor's appointment?" When I respond that way, people usually have no further comment. I have discovered that people don't really want to change unless they are forced to change due to an illness and that included me.

Many men and women know that good lifestyle choices, such as exercising regularly, eating a healthy diet, not smoking, and drinking in moderation make a big difference in staying healthy. But many have a hard time doing it and it is a shame that many often ignore these sensible recommendations until they've been diagnosed with a disease. Further, many people don't realize that environmental exposures can contribute to major diseases in addition to eating poorly and not exercising.

There has been significant research in recent decades showing that chronic conditions such as heart disease, prostate cancer, and infertility may be linked to everyday exposures to chemicals in water, consumer products, and food. There are lots of ways to reduce exposures to potentially harmful chemicals and other environmental risk factors, so why not decrease the chances and live the healthiest and longest life possible?

Real change takes desire

Our oldest son has a very hectic work life but he wanted to make a lifestyle change. His desire was to be healthier and in doing so he modified his schedule so he could exercise, eat healthier and juice. In the morning before work, he has a twelve to sixteen ounce green juice or smoothie and at lunch time he goes for a walk. Throughout the day he tries to eat as healthy as he can by eating more fruits and vegetables, organic meats, and follows the Mediterranean diet the best he can. After work he makes another green juice or smoothie. He also buys organic foods as much as possible or buys his produce and fruit from the farmer's market. Our youngest daughter has a busy, hectic work life as well, shops the same, and manages to cook most meals for her family of three boys. She wants to ensure they receive good nutritious food and instill in them healthy eating habits. In fact, most of our children have been trying to maintain a healthier lifestyle by eating healthier and organically as possible, exercising, and keeping a healthy weight. New behaviors can be customized to fit a daily schedule if there really is a desire to change.

Radical Remission

A change in attitude, I believe, helped save my life and changes like this are now bringing awareness to the medical community. In a recently published article in the "Breast Cancer Wellness" magazine by Kelly A. Turner, PhD wrote about Radical Remission.

Radical remission is not statistically expected. Radical remission is people who heal from cancer without using any conventional medicine, or people with cancer who first tried conventional medicine that did not work and switched to other methods that worked or people who use conventional and alternative medicine simultaneously to overcome a cancer prognosis of less than a 25% 5-year survival rate.

Turner maintains that some people credit these remissions as miracle healing by faith or religion or a spontaneous healing by chance. But she prefers the term "radical remission." Most people she studied ended up making radical changes to their lives and took offense at the idea that their healing was simply by accident. "Radical Remission" is people's radical changes that have led to a radical result, surviving cancer against all odds.

Turner was surprised to learn that people mainly spoke about managing their emotions and not about consuming vegetables and vitamins, which she expected. Survivors kept mentioning that releasing suppressed emotions such as stress, fear, grief, or resentment, helped them to heal their cancer. It was more about the power of letting go than the power of positive thinking because survivors don't have positive thoughts 100% of the time. But they do make it a priority to feel fully and then release fully any emotions that come to them whether it is positive or negative. They live fully in the present and in the moment, instead of being troubled by the past or worried about the future. This is what I believe about fear being false evidence appearing real.

Scientists now believe that the mind and body are not as separate as they once thought. They have learned that the connections between mind, brain, and immune systems interact with one another which come from releasing suppressed emotions. PNI (psycho-neuro-immunology) studies have shown that releasing suppressed emotions can boost the immune systems in a variety of ways, from increasing the Natural Killer (NK) cell activity to reducing tissue inflammation. In one study, breast cancer patients who took a ten week stress management course had higher white blood cell counts afterward, as compared to a control group of breast cancer patients who did not take the course. Finding a way to release the suppressed emotion of stress helped the women strengthen their immune systems which helped their body's to heal after a breast cancer diagnosis.

Be your own advocate

I will continue to do my own research and live by my decision for the rest of my life. I have lived past the one year I was given by all my doctors. Even though I felt pressured by doctors, particularly my oncologists to have chemotherapy treatments, I stayed steadfast to what I believed what was right for me and right for my body.

My general practitioner and my surgeons are kind of on board with me. They are not interested as to why I am doing so well instead they say, "Whatever you are doing keep doing it. It is working." My chiropractor is one of my best advocates. He had the opportunity to try the Gerson therapy himself while in medical school and because of his experience he understands what I go through on a daily basis. It has been helpful to compare our experiences. Many times he has given me and my husband suggestions and encouragement.

Being your own advocate is all about choosing how to take care of your body from this day forward. Eat good organic foods, juice when able, have good family support, and most of all *have a positive attitude*.

Chapter Sixteen

Knowledge is Important

JUST THINKING OF THE POSSIBILITY OF breast cancer, or any cancer for that matter, focuses the mind on fear and disease. Stress is actually enough to trigger an illness. It is well established in the medical community that stress has damaging effects on health. For those who have been recently diagnosed with cancer, the most important thing I can tell you is NOT TO PANIC! You probably feel you have been given the worst diagnosis in the world. Just this phrase, "You have cancer" will suddenly change your life forever and cloud your thinking. It is a rational fear. You may believe that your oncologist will save you because he or she has been trained at the best medical institutions and knows of the best available cancer treatments. But it is important to pay attention to what is being told to you so you fully understand it!

Ask questions, get answers

Be sure to ask your doctor as many questions as possible even if they seem irritated. Do not be intimidated just by their doctor status. It is your right to know all about your diagnosis and be informed. Write questions down as you think of them. In fact, write them down the minute they pop into your head before they are forgotten. Keep a paper and pen handy all the time because cancer and questions about it are the most prominent things on your mind. Have your list of questions ready before seeing your doctor and then make sure to write down the answers to your questions. My husband and I both wrote down answers to compare afterward. There is a tendency for one person to pick up what the other missed. Ask for a "nurse navigator" who can assist you with problems through the process. Navigators can be very helpful when the doctor is unavailable.

Be informed so you are able to *clearly* communicate with doctors regarding *your circumstance*. Not all remedies for cancer treatments are the same. I did my research before I made my decision. There are a lot of good doctors with good advice but take your time. Time is *not* of the essence! It is important to not let doctors, friends, or relatives frighten you into doing something you are not sure about or prepared to do. Try not to focus too much on any one thing by itself. Try and look at the whole picture as you think about your options. Be informed! Get informed! Inform others what you have learned! What I am saying here is that it is ok *not* to agree with doctors, friends, or relatives. They mean well and want to help, but after all, it's not their body. *Be comfortable with your decision and never regret the decision you made.*

If you have had surgery before being administered chemo, I recommend healing your body from the surgery first before you do anything else. That is what doctors want you to do anyway. Take the recovery time to research and figure out what you are going to be comfortable doing following your surgery. Then discuss your cancer treatment options with your doctor. If the doctors want you to do chemotherapy of any kind, research the kind they want to administer *before* you say yes and find out about all the side effects. There are hundreds of different kinds of chemotherapy with all kinds of side effects for all kinds of cancer. Visit www.chemocare.com, click on "drug information," and then click on the "drug name" they want to administer. The website will tell you a lot about the drug and its side effects. This site is fantastic and will help you understand chemotherapy.

I must affirm an important thing I learned about breast cancer surgery. If you had nodes removed, make sure you do not have blood pressure cuffs or blood testing done or anything that requires pressure such as tourniquets on the arm from which nodes were taken. If you are not careful and forget to tell the technician that lymph nodes were removed, it is possible to get lymphedema, a build-up of fluid that causes swelling in the arms or legs. This is a common side effect and can be painful. This information was not told to me by my doctors. I discovered this on my own and later asked one of my oncologists about it. The oncologist responded with, "Oh yes, this is important." There was no response when I asked why I wasn't told it. This is an example of why it is important to keep doing your own research!

Natural defense system

The reason there is cancer in a body is because the body's natural defense system is functioning poorly. It can take up to ten years before a tumor is detected. When a cancer cell shows up in a poorly functioning system, it cannot be destroyed. Nutritionally boosting the immune system or restoring it to a healthy state helps boost the body's natural defense system when there is a cancer diagnosis. Allopathic doctors (those with a traditional medical degree) do not include nutrition for boosting the immune system as part of a cancer treatment, especially as part of "standard" chemotherapies. Some foods can increase the growth and spread of cancer, but oncologists, in many cases, allow their patients to eat these types of foods, especially sugar. Sugar feeds every cell in our body—even cancer cells. In my experience with oncologists there seems to be a consensus to negate this fact. On one of my visits to my oncologist I saw bowls of candy on the counters of the lobby area. I noted my observation to my oncologist as I was leaving his office and asked why he had bowls of candy on the counters for cancer patients when it is known that sugar feeds cancer cells. I also stated I felt sugar should be removed from the cancer patient's diet. He preferred to stick to the fact that sugar does not cause cancer. I agreed that this was true and again said but sugar feeds it. His face became red, as it often did when I questioned why he did things, and no more was said. Surgery, drugs, and radiation is what has been taught in medical school and little is taught about nutrition.

Nutrition is a natural defense system and while it is starting to be talked about more, not enough is being done to educate patients about the importance of nutrition. Only thirty percent of medical schools in the U.S. require medical students to take a separate nutrition course. On average, students received 23.9 contact hours of nutrition instruction during medical school (range was 2 to 70 hours). Only 40 of 126 medical schools require the 25 hour minimum recommended by the National Academy of Sciences. Researchers at the School of Medicine of the University of North Carolina at Chapel Hill concluded that the amount of nutrition education in medical schools remains inadequate. With this in mind, it is important for you to know *you* need to help *your* body fight off recurring cancer cells by boosting your own immune system by eating properly to enhance the effectiveness of treatments.

Boosting the Immune System

In order to boost my immune system, I continue to juice and eat properly. Through integrative medicine resources, as discussed earlier, I receive intravenous, B-17 (laetrile) and vitamin C in high doses at least four times a year. Integrative medicine is the combination of practices and methods of alternative medicine with conventional biomedicine.

Intravenous vitamin C has been considered an integrative medical therapy for cancer since the 1970s, but don't confuse this with oral vitamin C which does not compare to the immediate effects of the heavy dose of the intravenous vitamin C. In its February 2014 issue, Health Day News stated that large doses of intravenous vitamin C have the potential to boost the immune system's ability to kill cancer cells, even with chemotherapy. But it's been hard to attract funding for further research.

There's no reason for pharmaceutical companies to fund vitamin C research and federal officials have been uninterested in plowing research dollars into the effort, especially since the Mayo Clinic published research stating "that vitamin C given intravenously (IV) has been touted to have different effects than vitamin C taken orally. However, until clinical trials are completed, it's premature to determine what role IV vitamin C may play in the treatment of cancer." It is my opinion that even though the Mayo Clinic said there have been positive results for vitamin C given intravenously, the pharmaceutical companies are not interested in furthering research dollars because it is not a drug that can be patented.

Laetrile (B17 is also known as amygdalin) therapy is one of the most popular and best known alternative cancer treatments. Conventional medicine condemns it as quackery and the vast majority of cancer information sites claim that laetrile is useless as a cancer treatment. This is because since the 1970s there has been a laetrile cover-up.

Dr. Kanematsu Sugiura, one of the Sloan-Kettering Cancer Centers oldest and leading research scientists as well as the original co-inventor of chemotherapy, did a secret study on laetrile and had unexpectedly positive results. Ralph W. Moss PhD, a young, eager science writer working for Sloan-Kettering Cancer Center reported back to his superiors what Dr. Sugiura had discovered and was told to not discuss Dr. Sugiura's study further. However, Dr. Moss ignored this advice and while working as a loyal employee at Sloan-Kettering was recruiting fellow employees to help anonymously leak information about the laetrile's ability to heal cancer to the American public. One doctor, Dr. Daniel Martin, upon discovering information was being leaked, deliberately mixed up the experiment on a final "blind" test and used the erroneous information that laetrile was not effective against cancer. Several doctors with Sloan-Kettering lied at a press conference about the positive effects of laetrile. They all lied about an effective treatment for cancer! Dr. Martin continued to lie and promoted chemotherapy as a better cure while also making fraudulent claims against the effectiveness of laetrile. [1]

Research into laetrile has not stopped from the time when it was buried forty years ago. Mercola.com recites recent studies that substantiate Dr. Kanematsu Sugiura's work in the early 1970s:

- February 2003: Amygdalin from *Prunus persica* seeds (peach pits) shows anti-tumor effects comparable to epigallocatechin gallate in green tea [2]

- August 2006: Amygdalin also induces apoptosis (cell death) in human prostate cancer cells [3]

- February 2013: Amygdalin induces apoptosis in human cervical cancer cells; authors conclude it may offer a new therapeutic option for cervical cancer patients [4]

- May 2013: Amygdalin inhibits renal fibrosis in chronic kidney disease; researchers conclude it is a "potent antifibrotic agent that may have therapeutic potential for patients with fibrotic kidney diseases" [5]

- August 2014: In a new German study, amygdalin dose-dependently reduced growth and proliferation of bladder cancer [6]

Although laetrile is very effective in high doses at stopping the spread of cancer, not a cure, it should be combined with an effective cancer diet in order for a patient to have much better healing results. Laetrile works by targeting and killing cancer cells and building the **immune system** to fend off future outbreaks of cancer. It uses two different methods for killing cancer cells. It involves a strict diet (as do some cancer treatments) and several supplements. However, you need to do your own research to maximize its benefits as it does not reverse damage to the non-cancerous cells due to cancer chemotherapy or radiation treatments.

The FDA in the 1970s banned laetrile supplements despite its proven effectiveness and it is almost impossible to obtain, even though it is a perfectly natural and safe supplement. Even more confusing and hard to understand is that the sources of laetrile, B17, are both the same, but B17 is legally available.

Laetrile is available over the Internet, either as apricot kernels or pills and in some cases in liquid form. It is a must to research reliable companies from the Internet. I eat a small handful of raw apricot kernels once in a while with my breakfast and morning juice as well as combine intravenously, the legal B-17 (laetrile) and vitamin C in high doses.

Cancer and my friend

I have a friend who was diagnosed with HER2 breast cancer a year after my diagnosis. She had a partial mastectomy with good margins. She had a ping pong sized tumor (a ping pong ball has a diameter of 3.8 cm) and two lymph nodes removed with no metastases in the nodes. She was not sure the stage of the cancer so we guessed because of the tumor size and that there was no cancer in her lymph nodes that the cancer would have been stage II. She did not know any further information.

HER2 breast cancer is a treatable cancer and my friend wanted to know more about what I did during my treatment. We discussed what I went through regarding surgery and what I chose to do. She asked if I could invite her and her husband to our house for dinner so he could see how we now eat. She wanted her husband to be able to ask us questions about what I learned, what kind of research I did, and my experiences. She asked if it was possible to do it before she committed to chemotherapy as she wanted to show her husband there were solutions other than chemotherapy.

A few days later they came over for dinner. We juiced before and after dinner and her husband complimented us on the good tasting dinner but said if there was some meat it would have been a better meal. We answered as many questions as they asked. My friend was eager and wanted to learn more and try what I was doing. Her husband, on the other hand, felt what we were doing was too difficult for their circumstances and didn't want to change their lifestyle. And, there was no way he was going to give up meat and become a vegetarian. I explained he didn't have to give up meat entirely but should consider changing to a Mediterranean diet lifestyle where he could have meat but on a more limited basis. He curled his upper lip and said he liked the way they ate.

My friend argued that she could change and that she did not want to do chemotherapy. No more was said. We were thanked for the dinner and they left. A week later my friend called me crying. She had decided to do the standard chemotherapy treatment because she felt pressured by her family, doctors, and friends and husband, who did not want to change their eating habits. She is my friend so I supported her decision. I will continue to help her *whenever she asks*.

After her first chemotherapy infusion she lost her hair. By the completion of her second chemotherapy infusion she had already experienced many side effects, including blood in her urine and stools, fatigued, loss of appetite, and weight loss. Most days she experienced great pain. Pain medication and antidepressants got her through those days. She also complained of having chemo brain.

What is chemo brain?

Here are just a few examples of what patients call chemo brain according to www.cancer.org:

- Forgetting things that they usually have no trouble recalling (memory lapses)
- Trouble concentrating (they can't focus on what they're doing, have a short attention span, may "space out")
- Trouble remembering details like names, dates, and sometimes larger events
- Trouble multi-tasking, like answering the phone while cooking, without losing track of one task (they are less able to do more than one thing at a time)
- Taking longer to finish things (disorganized, slower thinking, and processing)
- Trouble remembering common words (unable to find the right words to finish a sentence)

Doctors and researchers call chemo brain a "mild cognitive impairment." Most define it as being unable to remember certain things and having trouble finishing tasks or learning new skills. How long it lasts is a major factor in how much it affects a person's life. These kinds of brain problems can cause trouble at work and at home. People who notice problems with their thinking may feel even more upset if their doctors blame it on aging or act like it's nothing to worry about. It's distressing to wonder if you'll ever be able to do your job again or if you'll get lost on the way to a place you've been to dozens of times.

One day just before my friend's third infusion, she asked if I could take her to the clinic to have a blood cell booster shot. When I arrived, she was eating a peanut butter, jelly and Nacho Cheese Doritos sandwich (Doritos have powerful toxins with high doses of MSG and sodium). I advised her that a whole wheat peanut butter and jelly sandwich was okay but she should skip the Doritos. She then said that this was the first day in almost four weeks she felt like eating something other than Ensure and black coffee. Her doctor, ironically my former oncologist, said that Ensure would give her energy and boost her immune system. She said she had just ordered more to sustain her. I felt an obligation to tell her what I learned about Ensure and more about nutrition. I asked her to research Ensure before consuming any more of it. I suggested she try to eat healthier to boost her immune system as that would be more beneficial during chemotherapy treatments than Ensure.

Ensure

According to fackfood.com Ensure is a fake food that is nothing but sugar water. The top four ingredients in Ensure are: water, sugar, corn syrup, and maltodextrin.

1 Water – not bad, but you are paying a high price for water.
2 Sugar – also known as sucrose. Sugar is a refined carbohydrate. Sugar has been strongly linked to the promotion of diabetes, clinical depression, weight gain, obesity, and various nutritional deficiencies. It's also an acidic ingredient that promotes osteoporosis by forcing the body to leach minerals out of its bones in order to buffer the acidity of the sugar. Sugar puts extra stress on the pancreas and liver, and if consumed in large quantities over time, sugar can result in decreased insulin sensitivity.

3   Corn syrup – also a refined carbohydrate with an extremely high glycemic index value. Corn syrup (and especially high-fructose corn syrup) has been linked to diabetes, obesity, problems with blood sugar control and insulin sensitivity. Corn syrup is frequently used as a sweetener. It is the primary sweetener in soft drinks, which is one of the reasons why soft drinks so strongly promote obesity.

4   Maltodextrin – derived from corn. Maltodextrin is yet another refined carbohydrate that's high on the glycemic index list.

That's basically *three sweeteners and water*. Sugar feeds every cell in our body—even cancer cells. But oncologists do not believe that sugar feeds cancer or causes cancer to grow. However, research has shown that eating sugar doesn't necessarily *lead* to cancer.

After a year my friend was not doing well. She had no energy, was in constant pain, and developed lymphedema. She was tired, very negative, very depressed, and had constant infections. She had been told if she continued to lose weight she would be admitted to the hospital to be force fed. I sincerely feared for her life but decided I cannot force anyone to change. She must want to change herself to succeed in being healthy again.

Cancer and my cousin

My cousin was diagnosed, ironically also a year after my diagnosis, with the estrogen receptor [ER] 75%, progesterone receptor [PR] 25% breast cancer. She underwent a partial mastectomy with good margins and ten nodes were removed. The sentinel node tested positive for metastatic carcinoma consistent with the breast tumor with no extra-capsular spread. Nine auxiliary nodes were negative. The main breast tumor measured 3.0 x 1.8 x 1.4cm. Therefore her pathology report classified the cancer at stage II.

Prior to committing to chemotherapy treatments, my cousin called me. We spoke at great length about my cancer diagnosis and my treatment decision. I sent her a letter regarding my research. We both had our concerns about cancer because her older sister passed away several years prior from breast cancer. The more we spoke, the more we discovered how much cancer was in our family, most being on our maternal side.

Even though my cousin and I both tested negative for BRCA1 and BRCA2 cancer gene, we feel there must be an unidentified hereditary gene for cancer somewhere in our DNA.

My cousin decided to do chemotherapy and learned about foods that would help her fight cancer while going through her treatments. She posted a list of the foods on her refrigerator. Her wonderful husband supported her by eating the cancer fighting foods with her and helped prepare their meals together. They had a garden, ate nutritious whole plant-based foods, and ate organic meats as much as possible or meats her husband had hunted or fished.

Both my cousin and my friend were doing the same chemotherapy treatment and coincidently their treatments were a week apart from each other. When my cousin finished her second chemotherapy infusion she had to undergo a booster shot to boost the blood cells too. She had other side effects including some fatigue, loss of hair, and pain from the blood cell booster shot. Contrary to my friend's experiences, my cousin's symptoms were not as severe.

My cousin said each chemotherapy treatment had different symptoms and it was difficult for her to prepare for the next symptom but regardless she continued proper nutrition. After her radiation treatments she had painful moderate burns in her armpit area, minor burns to her breast, and fatigue. She was prescribed a cream medication for the pain and burn "discomfort" and healed fine. In spite of all this she remained active, positive, worked outside in her garden, and walked most days.

We kept in contact with each other through her treatments and gave each other support. My husband and I visited my cousin and her husband after her treatments were completed. I am happy to report that she looked great, continued to have a positive attitude, and made a cancer-free recovery. When I related my friend's side effects to my cousin, we were both convinced we did the right thing for our personal cancer treatment choices, which included a lifestyle change.

Although this experience is not a "scientific" study, it is one that has been personally observed. However, the three of us had strikingly different approaches to cancer. My cousin and I feel we had an advantage over my friend: family support, proper eating habits with nutritious cancer fighting foods, and a lifestyle change. My friend did not change her lifestyle and she continued to be ill. My cousin and I are convinced that these three elements are the most important parts of healing from our cancer diagnosis. The two of us continue to compare our findings with each other and are grateful for the knowledge we have learned, applied, and continue to apply.

My friend, my cousin and I were diagnosed with Stage II cancer and we all learned how debilitating cancer can be regardless what was chosen to combat it.

Chapter Seventeen

Healthy Diets

AFTER COMPLETING MY TWO YEARS of alternative therapy and being cancer free, I eat a modified Mediterranean diet, which is primarily vegetarian. Neither vegetarians nor vegans eat meat. However, vegetarians tend to consume dairy products and eggs while vegan avoids *all* animal products, including eggs and dairy.

The Mediterranean diet is a lifestyle not a short term fad diet. In his book *Health Via Food*, William Howard Hay wrote, "First let us get rid of this accepted idea that any modification of conventional habit in foods is diet, for the diet is a restriction of eating for some definite purpose, as the relief from some specific diseased state. What we mean here by diet is nothing of the kind, but merely a normalizing of the daily intake of foods to bring this measurably toward the ideal."

I continue to juice; however my juicing regimen is less now, two to four, twelve ounce juices daily depending on what I am doing and where I am going. I strive for at least one carrot/apple and two green juices a day to maintain a proper pH balance (pH balance will be described later in another chapter). When traveling, we search for organic juice bars and typically locate one or more in large metropolitan areas. It is far more difficult in rural areas.

Taking Charge

Changing the way we eat and taking charge of our bodies is critical. I recommend the Mediterranean diet as well as the Nordic diet, vegetarian diet and the Indian and Asian cuisines for a lifestyle change for those who are currently on the Standard American Diet (S.A.D.). These diets specifically can reduce inflammation in the body and promote a healthy disease fighting immune system.

The abbreviation for the Standard American Diet is S.A.D. because the average American eats a lot of food that is unhealthy. S.A.D. describes the stereotypical Western dietary pattern of Americans. It is a diet high in red meat, sugar, high-fat foods, and refined grains. It also includes high-fat dairy products, high-sugar drinks, and is high in processed meat.[1] Obviously, these foods are not healthy, yet Americans are still eating them. S.A.D. has been positively linked to obesity, death from heart disease, colon cancer, and breast cancer.[2] In order to regain their health Americans need to change. Americans need a lifestyle change and need to teach our children how to eat **by example and not by convenience**. Protect our children.

I first learned about the Mediterranean diet at The Longevity Center (TLC) could implement this diet after completing my two years of the Gerson Therapy if I desired. I was reminded of the diet again at the University of Stanford's Cancer Center. I now do a combination of the Mediterranean diet (traditional dietary patterns of Greece, Southern Italy, Croatia and Spain) and the Nordic diet (seasonal dietary patterns of Norway, Sweden and Denmark). Both the Mediterranean diet and the Nordic diet encourage people to eat less red meat and more fish and tend to lean toward eating more vegetables. I do not eat beef, pork, or poultry but I do eat fish once in a while and enjoy an occasional glass of red wine.

I am a cancer survivor and I believe I survived because I changed my lifestyle and I cannot emphasize strongly enough how important it is to maintain a healthy nourishing diet. Our ancestors didn't worry about heart disease, cancer, diabetes, Alzheimer's, or Parkinson's disease. They ate real food that nourished their bodies. We need to be vigilant to maintain the traditional foods that our ancestors ate (more nutrition per calorie) and veer from the non-nutritional foods that dominate our supermarkets today.

I agree with Nourishing Traditions, authors Sally Fallon and Mary G. Enig, Ph.D. that we should eat foods grown by independent producers of organic produce and grass-fed animals. I am suspicious of the powerful and highly profitable grain cartels, vegetable oil producers, and the food processing industry of the latest nutritional fad, pasteurized milk products and processed cheese. Fallon and Enig challenge politically correct nutrition such as "nutritional cookbooks" that follow politically correct guidelines, including all those approved by the American Heart Association.

In my opinion, a good example of a "bad politically correct nutrition" is the bestselling *Eater's Choice* by Dr. Ron Goor and Nancy Goor. It discusses studies that were said to implicate saturated fats as the cause of heart disease yet the book has many recipes loaded with refined sugar and refined white flour.

What we eat can either make our body stronger or rob us of vitality and energy. When we continue an unhealthy diet, over time our body will break down as our organs require more energy to digest the foods we eat. We will gain weight or become obese and more susceptible to diseases in the long run. Know and understand your body and utilize the Mediterranean diet properly. It can be modified to fit your body.

In this book, I focus on the Mediterranean diet, an alkalizing diet, because it is easier to follow for those who have a true desire to change their lifestyle and food choices.

According to the recommendations of the Mediterranean diet it emphasizes plant foods, fresh fruit as the typical daily dessert, olive oil as the main source of fat and dairy products such as cheese and yogurt. Fish and poultry should be consumed in low to moderate amounts and eggs should be no more than three per week and red meat should be consumed in lower amounts. Herbs and spices are used instead of salt to flavor foods. Wine can also be consumed in low to moderate amounts and the diet also requires regular physical activity.

The following is the Mediterranean diet from the Stanford's Cancer Center that could be utilized by most people who really want to improve their lifestyle regardless of any disease. Remember to use only organic products and know what your body can tolerate.

Mediterranean Diet

- Eat a variety of eight to ten servings of fruits, vegetables, and legumes and beans daily by following the seasons to broaden the range of nutrients you take in over the year.
- Vibrantly colored fruits and vegetables
- Increase cruciferous vegetables (broccoli, cauliflower, brussel sprouts and cabbage)
- Increase vegetables high in carotenoids (orange and dark green vegetables such as carrots, sweet potatoes and kale)

Consume a high fiber diet:

- Increase beans and whole grains (brown rice, oatmeal, and quinoa); whole grain breads and pastas must be GMO free to avoid pesticides. These are a great source of fiber and protein; nuts and seeds also provide healthy fats and antioxidants. Eat a serving of legumes (1/2 cup, cooked)—found in hummus or lentil soup—at least twice a week and a small portion of nuts daily (about one tablespoon, or ten to twelve almonds or walnut halves).
- Avoid processed and refined foods and grains (white flour and sugar). Refined carbohydrates lack nutrients and can spike blood sugars. Whole grains are best. Try pasta made from quinoa, rice or Jerusalem artichoke. Incorporate sprouted or fermented grains

like sourdough for easier digestion and better nutrient absorption.

Aim for a low fat diet:

- Limit saturated fats (butter, dairy, and animal fats)
- Avoid fried and barbecued foods cooked in fats that are solid at room temperature. These fats are typically saturated and raise the cholesterol more than anything else in the diet.
- Avoid fats such as margarines and shortenings, which are hydrogenated and are called trans-fats. (Use organic non-hydrogenated shortening substitute.)
- Include healthy fats (flax oil, hemp oil, canola oil, olive oil, avocado oil, raw avocados, nuts, and seeds)

Minimize animal proteins:

- Limit red meats to once every two weeks (beef, pork, lamb); grass fed or wild is better
- Limit poultry and eggs to three ounces once a week (each egg is one ounce)
- Avoid processed meats like salt-cured, smoked, and nitrate cured foods (bacon, sausage, pepperoni, and luncheon meats)

Consume healthy animal proteins:

- Eat three to four ounces of yogurt daily at least 30 minute before eating a meal or two hours after. Yogurt is a cultured dairy as well as kefir, fresh curd cheeses like ricotta. Cultured dairy is easier to digest and supplies beneficial bacteria that contribute to digestive health.
- Increase cold-water three ounce serving size of fish to twice a week (wild salmon, herring, tuna, sardines, black cod, sablefish, anchovies, and arctic char)

Limit consumption of salty foods:

- Avoid processed foods, especially those containing salt and additives. Add herbs and spices for flavor (rosemary, thyme, oregano, parsley, sage, ginger, turmeric, or garlic). They are full of plant compounds with antioxidants and have inflammation-fighting effects.

Limit alcohol consumption or don't drink at all:

- Red wine consumption can be three, three to five ounce servings per week. Red wine contains resveratrol, which is a potent anti-oxidant.

Healthy tea consumption:

- Drink one to four cups of green tea daily. Green tea seems to help keep blood sugar stable in people with diabetes as it contains catechins, which lower cholesterol as well as high blood pressure. Catechins are antioxidants that fight and may even prevent cell damage.

- Drink herbal teas made from herbs, fruits, seeds, or roots steeped in hot water (ginger, ginkgo biloba, ginseng, hibiscus, jasmine, rosehip, mint, rooibos (red tea), chamomile, and echinacea). Chamomile has antioxidants that may help prevent complications from diabetes, like loss of vision and nerve and kidney damage, and stunt the growth of cancer cells. Echinacea can fight the common cold and if you drink three cups of hibiscus tea daily can lower blood pressure in people with modestly elevated levels.

Limit calorie intake to achieve or maintain a healthy body weight.

- The body mass index (BMI) is one way to estimate a healthy weight. For most people it should vary between 18.5% and 24.9% depending on a person's overall weight. Higher and lower values are proportional to increased risk. It is estimated that obesity relates to 14% of cancer deaths in women. To calculate your BMI, divide your weight in pounds by your height in inches squared, and then multiply the results by a conversion factor of 703. For someone who is 5 feet 5 inches tall (65 inches) and weighs 150 pounds, the calculation would look like this: $[150 \div (65)^2]$ x $703 = 24.96$.

Mediterranean Diet Pyramid

A contemporary approach to delicious, healthy eating

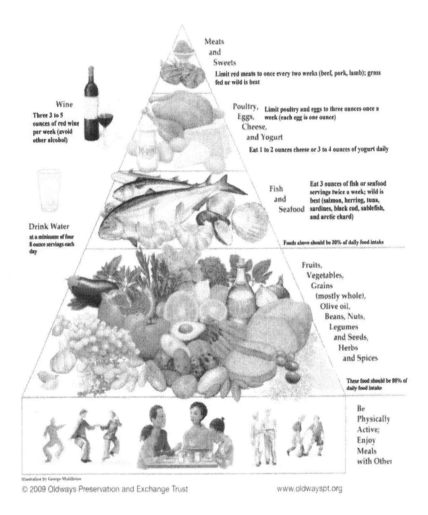

Meats and Sweets
Limit red meats to once every two weeks (beef, pork, lamb); grass fed or wild is best

Wine
Three 3 to 5 ounces of red wine per week (avoid other alcohol)

Poultry, Eggs, Cheese, and Yogurt
Limit poultry and eggs to three ounces once a week (each egg is one ounce)
Eat 1 to 2 ounces cheese or 3 to 4 ounces of yogurt daily

Fish and Seafood
Eat 3 ounces of fish or seafood servings twice a week; wild is best (salmon, herring, tuna, sardines, black cod, sablefish, and arctic chard)

Drink Water
at a minimum of four 8 ounce servings each day

Foods above should be 20% of daily food intake

Fruits, Vegetables, Grains (mostly whole), Olive oil, Beans, Nuts, Legumes and Seeds, Herbs and Spices

These food should be 80% of daily food intake

Be Physically Active; Enjoy Meals with Other

Illustration by George Middleton

© 2009 Oldways Preservation and Exchange Trust

www.oldwayspt.org

A handout from the Stanford Cancer Center and The Longevity Center

Nordic Diet

"Move over Mediterranean diet, the traditional Nordic diet could be key to losing weight" says Dietitians Association of Australia (DAA) spokesperson Georgie Rist. According to Rist the Nordic diet places more emphasis on nutrient-dense foods that have been grown in the wild and on seasonal, organic produce. It's not so different from the Mediterranean diet in the sense that it promotes moderate consumption of fat, protein, and antioxidant-packed ingredients. What olive oil, nuts, beans, and sardines are to the Mediterranean diet, canola oil, berries, root vegetables, and cod are to the Nordic diet.

In Australia, the levels of chemical residue in food are regulated, so all food is safe to eat, regardless of whether or not it's organic. Both organic and conventionally-grown produce can provide all the nutrients required if a healthy, balanced diet is followed. It is my opinion that America needs to promote Australia's type of growing! Americans are being poisoned from all the cancer-causing pesticides and GM products allowed in farming.

The philosophy of sustainable, seasonal eating is also one that is being embraced by Scandinavian chefs. The Danes complained of how difficult it was to integrate healthy Mediterranean foods into their regular diet because of the cost and availability of transported foods. Therefore the Nordic diet was created in 2004 by a group of nutritionists, scientists and chefs, in order to address growing obesity rates and unsustainable farming practices in the Nordic countries. The key theme of the Nordic diet was to ensure that only local and in-season foods were chosen.[3]

Thomas Meinert Larsen, Ph.D., conducted and led a study in Denmark with a group of people on the Nordic diet and a group who followed an average Danish diet (pasta, bread, pizza, potatoes, and rice and dairy products). Both groups were allowed to eat as much as they wanted and could deviate from the prescribed plan occasionally, though all food intake was monitored. Dr. Larson found that those who had generally followed the Nordic diet had eaten fewer calories each day over a six-month period and said: "Our view is that eating foods in accordance with the seasons makes us less dependent on transportation. There's particular emphasis on foraged foods because they taste better, and usually contain greater amounts of vitamins and minerals than conventionally grown plants."[3]

In his study, Dr. Larsen also found that the overweight participants who ate the new Nordic diet lost three times as much weight as their counterparts who stuck to the ordinary Danish diet. The mean weight change was a loss of 10.3 pounds for the Nordic diet group and a loss of 3.3 pounds for the Danes diet group. Further, the Nordic diet produced greater reductions of systolic and diastolic blood pressure, than the ordinary diet.

Dr. Larsen noted that the concept of a healthy, regional, sustainable, seasonal and tasty diet could in principle be applied anywhere in the world, not just Nordic countries. He suggested that in time that it could challenge the Mediterranean diet for the title of world's healthiest diet.

The Nordic diet is simple and easy to follow as it is not much different than the Mediterranean diet which has been embraced by the Western medical community as a healthy lifestyle diet.

How to Eat Nordic

- *Less Red Meat More Fish:* Both the Mediterranean Diet and the Nordic Diet emphasize eating less red meat. If red meat is eaten, it should be high quality, lean organic or wild meat. Georgie Rist says that omega-3 oily fish should be increased because it "will increase healthy omega-3 fats and decrease your levels of unhealthy saturated fats, and Omega-3s are important for our heart, brain, joints, eyes, mood and nervous system."[4] The average national intake of omega-3s in America is 246 milligrams per day far below the recommendation of 610 milligrams a day for men and 430 milligrams for women.

- *Snack on Berries:* Choose red and purple berries, in particular, as these are high in antioxidants, the natural plant compounds that offer protection from cancer, heart disease, and strokes.

- *Eat Rye Bread:* Rye bread is a Nordic staple, and Rist says it's one of the best grain sources of fiber available. "It contains approximately three times more fiber than white wheat bread. Rye is also rich in magnesium, B vitamins, iron, zinc, phytochemicals, and antioxidants."[4] Rye promotes a feeling of fullness, so it can help with weight loss. It also helps manage blood sugars and cholesterol levels and promotes a healthy bowel.

- *Eat More Root Vegetables:* Because of cold climate, Scandinavians eat lots of potatoes and root veggies which grow in cooler temperatures. Potatoes and fleshy enlarged root vegetables such as carrots, rutabaga, or beets are an excellent source of fiber, magnesium and potassium, says Rist.[4]

- *Use Oils Low in Saturated Fats:* The Nordic cooking oil staple is canola, as it's manufactured from a cool-climate crop (rapeseeds). It's low in saturated fat but rich in heart-healthy monounsaturated fats. A similar fat ratio, such as extra-virgin olive oil, is also good for heart health and wellbeing.

The University of Copenhagen developed a number of principles which now form the basis of a New Nordic Diet developed in 2004. It is considered "new" because many of the foods on the "ordinary Nordic" diet were actually never eaten in the Nordic countries back in the day. The new principles resulted in a list of basic ingredients for the New Nordic Diet as well as recommendations as to dietary intake.

Principles of the Diet

1. Eat more fruit and vegetables often (berries, cabbage, root vegetables, legumes, potatoes, and herbs, spices and rapeseed (canola) oil.

2. Eat more whole grains, nuts and seeds often (especially rye, oats, and barley)

3. Eat more food from the seas and lakes (fish and seafood)

4. Rarely eat red meats and animal fats (higher quality meats and game meats, free-range eggs, cheese and yogurt)

5. Eat more food from wild landscapes
6. Eat organic produce where possible
7. Avoid food additives (sugar-sweetened beverages, added sugars, processed meats, and refined fast foods)
8. Eat more meals that are based on seasonal produce
9. Eat more meals that are home-cooked and less restaurant foods
10. Produce less waste

The Nordic diet emphasizes locally grown and sustainable food sources, with a heavy focus on foods considered healthy as listed above. However, being healthy requires devotion to health. According to the data gathered by the World Health Organization, in 2007 "Just 5.8 percent of women in Norway are considered to be significantly overweight, making its people among the slimmest in the developed world." [5] The reasons are simple. They walk, jog or ride bikes instead of driving. Kids grow up hiking and skiing, veer from sugar and junk foods, but most importantly, Norwegians teach children nutrition and promote healthy behavior that impact modern life and put emphasis on family meals, cooking and eating together.[5]

The Nordic diet is actually very similar to the Mediterranean diet with the biggest difference emphasizing canola/rapeseed oil instead of extra virgin olive oil. Lately olive oil has come under scrutiny and label reading is a must to ensure you stay healthy.

In September 2013 the U.S. International Trade Commission, released a report—"Olive Oil: Conditions of Competition between U.S. and Major Foreign Suppler Industries"—evidence of rampant fraud was found.

"The United States does not have mandatory testing, nor does it impose penalties for noncompliance. This lack of enforcement has resulted in a long history of fraudulent practices (adulteration and mislabeling) in the olive oil sector." [6]

In the June 19, 2013 Consumer Reports News it was found that only 9 of the 23 olive oils from Italy, Spain and California tested, passed as being extra virgin olive oil even though all of them claimed so on the label.

"Olive oil marketers aim to differentiate their products by brand and level of quality, but price remains one of the most important factors in U.S. consumer purchasing decisions. This is due, in part, to a lack of consumer awareness of quality differences. U.S. consumers are generally unfamiliar with the range of olive oil grades and uses". [6]

What is Extra Virgin Olive Oil?

- Oil must come from fresh olives that were milled within 24 hours of their harvest
- Oil must be extracted by mechanical means (cold-pressed), not from heat or chemicals
- Oil must not be treated chemically in any way
- Extra virgin oil is in fact fresh olive juice
- Olives are a fruit which contain natural antioxidants that protect the plant during its lifetime. When the olive tree is very old it contains more of these antioxidants. This is one of the reasons that olive trees are often hundreds of years old and create anti-oxidant rich products. [7]

In July 2010 the UC Davis Olive Center issued a report showing that 69 percent of imported olive oils labeled as "extra virgin" failed the IOC sensory standard — in other words, these oils were defective and failed to meet the international standard for extra virgin olive oil. In the months since the release of the study, similar quality problems have been found in Andalusia, the world's most productive olive oil region, by Spanish authorities. In the same report, 83 percent of the imported samples that failed the IOC/USDA sensory standards also failed the German/Australian 1,2-diacylglycerol content (DAGs) standard. Two additional imported samples that met the IOC/USDA sensory standard for extra virgin failed the DAGs standard. [8]

Tips to recognize real Extra Virgin Olive Oil from altered oil

1. Ensure that the oil is labeled "extra virgin," since other categories—"pure" or "light" oil, "olive oil" and "olive pomace oil" — have undergone chemical refinement. Light olive oil or a blended olive oil isn't virgin quality.
2. Inexpensive extra virgin olive oil may not be real.
3. Olive oil in dark bottles protects the oil from oxidation and is a sign it is real olive oil.
4. Real extra virgin olive oil must have the International Olive Oil Council (IOC) seal.
5. Read the harvesting date on the label for freshness.
6. Real extra virgin olive oil will become thick and cloudy as it cools completely in the refrigerator. However, some oils made from high-wax olive varieties may solidify so all the tips must be verified to ensure it is real extra virgin olive oil.

These olive oils have met the extra-virgin standards:

- Corto Olive Oil
- Kirkland Toscano (Costco's brand)
- Kirkland Organic (Costco's brand)
- Cobran Estate Olive Oil (Australia's most awarded extra virgin olive oil)
- California Olive Ranch
- Lucero (Ascolano)
- McEvoy Ranch Organic
- Ottavio and Omaggio are good oils at reasonable prices
- Whole Foods California 365 olive oils [7]

The main type of fat found in olive oil is monounsaturated fatty acids (MUFAs). MUFAs are actually considered a healthy dietary fat. Replacing saturated and trans-fats with unsaturated fats such as MUFAs and polyunsaturated fats (PUFAs) may have certain health benefits.

According to the Mayo Clinic, MUFAs and PUFAs may help lower the risk of heart disease by improving related risk factors. For instance, MUFAs have been found to lower total cholesterol and low-density lipoprotein (LDL) cholesterol levels. MUFAs may also help normalize blood clotting. And some research shows that MUFAs may also benefit insulin levels and blood sugar control, which can be especially helpful in type II diabetes.

Find the right olive oil and stay healthy.

Chapter Eighteen

Eating with pH in Mind

EATING AN ALKALIZING DIET CAN help the body become beautiful and healthy. Consuming a meal that makes up an alkalizing environment with healthy pH levels between 6.0-7.5 levels can be easily done. But most Americans are not eating the right diet that produces an alkaline body. In fact, a large percentage of the world's population thinks that they are eating healthily but in reality we have been misled by the media and government on what is healthy and what is not.

To stop having exhaustion and chronic health problems that bother you every single day of your life, the diet has to change. Being heavy and feeling lethargic is caused by excessive fats in the body. Stop the body from creating these symptoms and reacting to an acidic diet.

In order for a body to be healthy it needs proper nutrients, minerals, trace minerals and enzymes. To restore its health, the body needs the power of nature, with 80 percent being vegetables and fruit and lots of hydration. Hydration should be a minimum of eight 8 ounce glasses of water or juice each day. If you like water with meals, it's best to drink a room-temperature water as ice water slows digestion. Caffeine drinks such as coffee, teas, and colas, along with alcoholic beverages have a diuretic effect that causes the body to eliminate more water and therefore, should be avoided. Foods containing the proper pH levels help the body to heal.

Acid Alkaline Imbalance

It is very common today that over acidity in the body can be a dangerous condition that weakens all the body's systems and can cause disease. A body with the proper pH balanced environment allows the normal body functions to resist disease and meet emergency demands. The body is weakened when the excess acids are not neutralized which cause the alkaline reserves to be depleted. According to many experts, a pH balanced diet is a vital key to health maintenance and alkalizing the body tissues can boost overall health and the health of specific areas of the body.

In 1933 a New York doctor, William Howard Hay, published *A New Health Era* in which he maintains that all disease is caused by self-poisoning due to acid accumulation in the body and that health problems are caused by the wrong chemical condition in the body. He explains: "Now we depart from health in just the proportion to which we have allowed our alkalies to be dissipated by introduction of acid-forming food in too great amount... It may seem strange to say that all disease is the same thing, no matter what its myriad modes of expression, but it is verily so."

In a book *Alkalize or Die*, written by Theodore A. Baroody. MA, DC, ND, L.M.T., PhD a nutritionist, says essentially the same thing: "The countless names of illnesses do not really matter. What does matter is that they all come from the same root cause...too much tissue acid waste in the body!"

Understanding pH

pH (potential of hydrogen) is a measurement of the acidity or alkalinity of a solution. The pH scale can tell if a liquid is more acid or more base, just as the Fahrenheit or Celsius scale is used to measure temperature. The range of the pH scale is from 0 to 14 from very acidic to very basic. A pH of 7 is neutral. A pH less than 7 is acidic and a pH greater than 7 is basic—the lower the pH the more acidic the solution, the higher the pH the more alkaline (or base) the solution. When a solution is neither acid nor alkaline it has a pH of 7 which is neutral.

Water is made up of hydrogen and oxygen and is the most abundant compound in the human body. The body is 70% water and has an acid-alkaline (or acid-base) ratio called the pH. The pH is a balance between positively charged ions (acid-forming) and negatively charged ions (alkaline-forming.) When the pH balance is compromised many problems can occur. Have you ever had an overactive acid problem in your stomach caused by overeating or eating the wrong foods? If so you probably took a commercial preparation intended to neutralize the acid in your stomach such as Alka-Seltzer or bicarbonate sodas which are alkaline products. However, it is important to understand that we are not talking about stomach acid or the pH of the stomach, but pH imbalance may cause these problems. We are talking about the pH of the body's fluids and tissues which is an entirely different matter.

People who suffer from a pH imbalance are acidic. Acidity forces the body to borrow minerals including calcium, sodium, potassium, and magnesium from vital organs and bones to neutralize the acid and safely remove it from the body. This strain on the body can cause severe and prolonged damage due to high acidity which may go undetected for years.

Mild acidosis can cause such problems as:

- Cardiovascular damage, including the constriction of blood vessels and the reduction of oxygen
- Weight gain, obesity, and diabetes
- Bladder and kidney conditions, including kidney stones
- Immune deficiency
- Acceleration of free radical damage, possibly contributing to cancerous mutations
- Hormone concerns
- Premature aging

- Osteoporosis; weak, brittle bones, hip fractures and bone spurs
- Joint pain, aching muscles and lactic acid buildup
- Low energy and chronic fatigue

Testing Acidity or Alkalinity with pH Strips in the Body

Using pH test strips can give immediate results and the pH factor can quickly and easily be analyzed at home. pH is determined by immersing the strip in the liquid to be tested and comparing its color with a standard color chart provided with the pH strip. If the urinary pH fluctuates between 6.0 and 6.5 in the morning and between 6.5 and 7.0 in the evening, the body is functioning within a healthy range. If the saliva pH stays between 6.5 and 7.5 all day, the body is functioning within a healthy range. In most cases strips are used either for urine or saliva and can be purchased on-line or through the local drug store.

pH Urine testing may indicate how well the body is eliminating acids and assimilating minerals, especially calcium, magnesium, sodium, and potassium. These minerals function as "buffers" that help maintain and balance the body against too much acidity or too much alkalinity. Acid or alkaline levels can become too high even with proper buffer amounts and the body must expel the excess through the urine. If the urine pH is below 6.5 the body is overwhelmed and "autotoxication" exists which is a sign that acid levels should be lowered.

Saliva testing results may indicate the activity of digestive enzymes in the body. Enzymes are primarily manufactured by the stomach, liver, and pancreas. Saliva also utilizes buffers just like urine, but to a lesser degree. If the saliva pH is too low, below 6.5, the body may be producing too many acids and has lost the ability to adequately remove them through the urine. If the saliva pH is too high, over 6.8, the body may suffer from too much gas, constipation, yeast infections or fungus. Some people will have acidic pH readings from both urine and saliva—"double acid" test.

Follow an alkaline diet and start using food to heal the body and lose weight naturally. With the application of the acid/alkaline principles, the daily dietary habits and lifestyle can lead to a healthy alkalized pH level the body requires.

The Mediterranean and Nordic Diets are Alkaline Diets and will help to:

- Improve the digestion system by reducing the amount of acidic food that is stuck in the stomach for the entire day
- Help to become more focused, promote mental clarity and renewed vigor as a result of balancing the pH level in the blood
- Get rid of chronic health issues like rashes, acid reflux, Gastroesophageal reflux disease (GERD), high blood pressure, arthritis, cancer, and other degenerative diseases by just eating the right alkalizing foods

In the pH Balance table, on the following page, it is important to note that a food's acid or alkaline forming tendency in the body has nothing to do with the actual pH of the food itself. For example, lemons are very acidic; however after digestion and assimilation, very alkaline. Therefore, lemons are alkaline forming in the body. The same is true for meat. Meat will test alkaline before it is digested but it is very acidic in the body after digestion. Like nearly all animal products, meat is very acid forming, which is why a vegetable rich diet and less meat are healthier.

America, Wake Up!

pH Balance TABLE

Acidic Range			Human Body pH Range		Alkaline Range	
4.0 - 5.0 most acidic	5.0 - 6.0 more acidic	6.0 - 7.0 acidic	7.0 neutral	7.0 - 8.0 alkaline	8.0 - 9.0 more alkaline	9.0 - 10.0 most alkaline
			water			
Dasani, Aquafina Distilled, Purified Vitamin Water	Dannon Springs Crystal Springs	Hawaii Water	Most municipal tap Supermarket spring water is +7.0	Fiji Whole Foods 365 Eden Springs	Trinity Sole	Ionized Water
			food categories			
Blue Berries Cranberries Prunes Sweetened Fruit Juice	Canned fruits Sour cherries Rhubarb	Plums Processed fruit juices	FRUITS	Oranges, Bananas Cherries, Pineapple Peaches, Avocados	Dates, Figs, Melons Grapes, Kiwi, Berries Pear, Apple, Raisins	Lemons, Limes Watermelon Grapefruit, Mango Papaya
Chocolate	Potatoes (no skins), Pinto, Navy, Lima, Split pea, Green pea Chickpea, Peanut	Cooked Spinach, Black eyed peas Kidney, Fava White beans	VEGETABLE BEAN LEGUME	Carrots, Tomatoes, Beets, Sweet Corn, Eggplant, Peas, Mushrooms, Lentils, Cabbage, Olives Potatoes (with skin)	Squashes, Yams, Green beans, Okra, Celery, Lettuce, Sweet Potato, Zucchini, Carob	Sea weeds, Onion, Kale, Cultured Vegetables, Parsley, Asparagus, Garlic, Raw Spinach, Endive, Spirulina, Broccoli
Pork, Beef Shellfish Pheasant Canned Tuna	Turkey Chicken Lamb	Venison Cold water fish, Liver Wild duck	MEATS			
Cheese, Custard Milk, Ice Cream Parmesan Hard Cheeses	Eggs, Butter Cottage Cheese Yogurt (processed)	Raw milk Whole milk	EGGS DAIRY	Goat cheese, Goat milk Whey Buttermilk Duck eggs	Kefir Soured milks Breast milk	
		Corn oil	OILS	Canola Cod liver	Flax oil, Ghee Primrose Avocado Pumpkin	Olive oil
White flour Pastries Pasta	White rice Corn meal Bread	Sprouted wheat Whole wheat Brown rice, Oat Rye, Barley	GRAINS CEREALS	Millet Amaranth Quinoa Buckwheat		
Peanuts Walnuts	Pecans Cashews Pistachios	Pumpkin Sesame Sunflower Pine nuts	NUTS AND SEEDS	Chestnuts Brazil Coconut	Hazelnut Almond Pumpkin	Poppy seeds
Liquor, Beer (Colas, Soft Drinks have pH of 3.0 and lower!)	Coffee Wine Black tea	Cocoa Packaged juice	BEVERAGES	Ginger tea Most herbal teas	Fresh fruit juice Green tea Almond milk	Kombucha Green drinks Fresh vegetable juice Wheat grass
	White sugar Brown sugar	Processed honey	SWEETENERS	Raw honey Raw sugar	Mayple syrup Rice syrup Black strap molasses	Stevia
Table salt White vinegar	Catsup Mayonnaise Mustard	Balsamic vinegar Rice vinegar	SALT SEASONING VINEGAR	Tamari Nama Shoyu Umeboshi vinegar	Most herbs Seasonings Apple cider vinegar	Himalayan crystal salt Sea salt

← More Cooked   More Raw →

http://www.morealivenow.com/wp-content/uploads/2013/01/pH_01.gif

Chapter Nineteen

Establishing and Maintaining Habits

ACCORDING TO THE AMERICAN HEALTH Association more than one in three adults has some form of cardiovascular disease. The good news is 80 percent of heart disease and stroke can be prevented. Protect yourself from heart disease, which is the number one killer, and lower your risk of other diseases and improve your health. The goal is to establish and make a habit exercising and choosing foods that are nutritious and healthful. You can improve your cholesterol and blood pressure by exercising regularly and limiting saturated fat, and avoiding too many animal products such as red meats and full-fat dairy.

The desire to change from the S.A.D. lifestyle to a better lifestyle must be driven by something that is deep inside you. Is it just for you or the entire family, which may be something to think about too? Is it a true desire to be healthy? Know why you want to change and understand it. It is also important to understand that maintenance is different from just losing weight while achieving a new lifestyle. Losing weight comes naturally with proper eating habits and can be based on your diet alone. However to maintain weight loss, physical activity is an absolute must.

Do You Need Support?

Maybe you are the type of person that needs support before doing exercises. Everybody needs some emotional support once in awhile. Or perhaps you just need someone to help you stay accountable. If someone else in your family or a friend or co-worker is also looking for support, team up.

Are You Exercising?

According to Webmd.com people who have lost an average of 66 pounds and kept it off an average of 5.5 years, did so by moving for about an hour each day. You don't have to join a gym. Start small by incorporating physical activity into your daily routine a little more each day. Take the stairs instead of the elevator, park at the farthest end of the parking lot or use your lunch break to take a quick walk. Exercise doesn't have to be done all at once. If walking is your preferred method of exercise, break it up to 30 minutes in the morning and 30 minutes in the evening or afternoon. A good way to make sure you are walking fast enough is if you cannot talk normally while walking. In other words, your talking is labored and you need to breathe deeply and talk less.

Do something you enjoy. Maybe it's yoga or even a serious daily workout. Experiment to find out what exercise will work for you. The point is just moving 60 minutes a day will help. A way to make time for exercise is to watch less TV. The average American watches 28 hours of TV per week. Studies show 62% of people in the National Weight Control Registry who have all lost 30 pounds or more and kept it off for at least a year, watched 10 or fewer hours per week.

Are You Eating Breakfast?

One theory about weight loss and diet maintenance is that eating breakfast, not only is the most important meal of the day, but it sets the tone for the rest of your day. According to the American Dietetic Association, people who eat breakfast perform better in the school and work and have better concentration, problem-solving skills, and eye-hand coordination. Breakfast provides you with the energy and nutrients that lead to increased concentration. Studies show that breakfast can be important in maintaining a healthy body weight, can reduce hunger throughout the day, and help people make better food choices at other meals. Start out with something that gives you nutrition like a bowl of oatmeal topped with fruit and nuts, or low-fat yogurt with berries and granola, or an omelet loaded with veggies and some rye toast on the side. If you are in a hurry, make a breakfast smoothie with a banana, yogurt, nuts, soaked rolled oats, a half an avocado and a little organic maple syrup for a sweetener.

Is Your Diet Rich in Fiber?

Fiber comes from plant-based foods like vegetables, fruits, whole grains, beans, nuts, and legumes. Fiber helps you feel full which makes you less likely to overeat. Most Americans don't get enough of it. It has been proven that people who eat plenty of fiber, get regular physical activity, eat fewer calories, and watch the scale are more likely to succeed at long-term weight maintenance.

Are You Watching the Scale?

It is a good idea to weigh yourself regularly. When the University of Minnesota researchers monitored the scale habits of 1,800 dieting adults, they found that those who weighed themselves daily lost an average of 12 pounds over 2 years; weekly scale watchers lost only 6. The once-a-day group also was less likely to regain weight loss. I weigh myself every morning so I can monitor what I eat if I have gained weight. Have a plan for what to do if your weight exceeds the level you want it to be and act fast. If you see your weight starting to climb, think about reducing your food portions or skip dessert more often. Or if you stopped your 60 minute daily workout plan, you may need to get moving again.

Are You Staying the Course?

No one eats according to plan all the time, especially when on vacation or on a business trip. In fact it's almost impossible to keep eating healthy and stay on your weight loss goals when you are not on your regular routine. Vacations or business trips can be an excuse to live it up by eating rich foods that are not normally eaten. Restaurant foods usually have larger proportions and are often high in calories, fat, saturated fat, cholesterol, and sodium and low in fiber. But don't fret, it is OK. The trick is to get back on course as soon as possible. The secret is to choose foods wisely, eat in moderation, and stay as active as possible during your trip. It may be a good idea to investigate your eating options before you go. Email or call the concierge of your hotel and ask for restaurant suggestions. When I visit a new city I look up vegetarian friendly restaurants online to see what their menu choices are. Make it a learning experience, not a failure. Winston Churchill once said "Success is not final, failure is not fatal; it is the courage to continue that counts." Remember that you can move on from setbacks. It is the long haul and changes are not going to happen overnight. It is a lifestyle of good habits. Eat better and choose a diet lifestyle suitable for you.

Have you Stopped Smoking?

It's time to kick the habit. According to the American Health Association going smoke-free can help prevent not only heart disease and stroke, but also cancer and chronic lung disease. The payoff is almost immediate. Quit smoking and you'll have the same risk level for developing heart disease as non-smokers within only a few years.

Do You Know About Resveratrol?

Resveratrol can be important for your health and should be taken seriously in your diet as health maintenance. Resveratrol is part of a group of plant compounds called polyphenols which have antioxidant properties that protect the body against increased risk of cancer and heart disease. Early evidence shows that applying a gel containing resveratrol to the face might reduce the severity of acne and suggests that taking a resveratrol supplement in combination with vitamin C, zinc, and flavonoids slightly reduces coughing and mucus production in people with COPD. It can also reduce low-density lipoprotein (LDL) —the "bad" cholesterol—and prevents blood clots and inflammation. Chronic inflammation has been linked to numerous chronic diseases.

Resveratrol might be a key ingredient in red wine that helps prevent damage to blood vessels. According to the Mayo Clinic, while the health news about red wine might make it seem like a great addition to enjoy with an evening meal, doctors are wary of encouraging anyone to drink alcohol. That's because too much alcohol can have many harmful effects on the body. Still, many doctors agree that something in red wine appears to help the heart.

According to an article from www.mercola.com by Dr. Joseph M. Mercola, DO, resveratrol is found in grapes, which produce it as a defense against fungi. Muscatine grapes actually have the highest concentration of resveratrol in nature because of their extra thick skins and numerous seeds, where the resveratrol is concentrated. Concord grapes, along with other dark-skinned grapes are a resveratrol antioxidant super food. But there are other sources out there, including peanuts, pistachios, blueberries, cranberries, and even cocoa, dark chocolate (chocolate must be at least 80% cocoa, which contains less sugar and has more resveratrol). The plants from these foods make resveratrol to fight fungal infection, ultraviolet radiation, stress, and injury.

Resveratrol is unique among antioxidants because it can help protect the brain and nervous system, and studies show that its benefits for your health are wide reaching, including:

- Protecting cells from free radical damage
- Inhibiting the spread of cancer, especially prostate cancer
- Lowering blood pressure
- Keeping the heart healthy and improving elasticity in the blood vessels
- Normalizing the anti-inflammatory response
- Helping to prevent Alzheimer's disease

Because resveratrol appears to be so effective at warding off many diseases associated with aging, it is often referred to a "fountain of youth" that can extend lifespan. Keep resveratrol foods in your diet to assist in health maintenance.

Vitamin Supplements:

Vitamins should be combined with your diet to maintain and improve your health. Remember to bring vitamin supplements with you while on vacation or on business trips. Dr. Russell Blaylock wrote *Natural Strategies for Cancer Patients* which speaks earnestly about vitamin supplements and nutrition. It is important to understand which supplements are healthy, especially for those who are dealing with cancer. Always try to use the form of supplements that most closely resembles the ones found in nature or those that have been known to have anticancer effects. The following are Dr. Blaylock's recommendations for the use of certain supplements.

Carotenoids found in certain plants and fruits that are red, orange or yellow serve as antioxidants and are a good source of vitamin A. Some allopathic (conventional) doctors state that an overdose of vitamin A can be harmful. That is true if it is consumed in supplements and not by juicing or eating these types of food.

Vitamin E comes in a gelatin capsule mixed with oil, which is usually soybean oil. Soy mimics estrogen and has been known to promote cancer growth and should be avoided. Never use vitamin E acetate as it is poorly absorbed and can cause problems with the liver and has very little anticancer effect. The most powerful form of vitamin E is vitamin E succinate. It is a white powder in a capsule.

Use vitamin C ascorbate rather than ascorbic acid. Ascorbic acid may cause stomach upset and cannot be absorbed well. High doses of ascorbic acid cause acid buildup and increase the risk of osteoporosis. Magnesium ascorbate and calcium ascorbate are the best in fighting osteoporosis. When vitamin C is taken, vitamin E should also be taken as they work well together. All nutrients interact in the body and this is especially true when dealing with cancer. It has been found that vitamin E reduces the risk of breast cancer and when selenium is added to the vitamin E, the risk reduces even more.

Selenium has attracted attention because of its antioxidant properties. It is a mineral found in soil, water, and some foods and is required in trace amounts for normal health, and is an essential element. The selenium antioxidants protect cells from damage. There is some evidence that selenium supplements may reduce the odds of prostate cancer. It is a safe mineral supplement and the general recommendation is 200 mcg a day. The safest limit for selenium is 400 micrograms (mcg) a day in adults. Anything above that is considered an overdose. Cancer patients should NOT take selenomethionine because of the methionine. Methionine is an amino acid that aids the liver in processing fats and it may cause conditions including recurrent bladder infections. Therefore, selenomethionine is not recommended for cancer or Parkinson disease patients. However, the body can typically meet the need for this nutrient through diet and would unlikely require supplementation for this purpose. The best source is *selenium-enhanced garlic.*

CoQ10 is a powerful nutrient and antioxidant that is a supplier of cellular energy and a cancer preventative. Cancer patients taking medicines must pay attention to CoQ10. Some medicines lower the body's supply of CoQ10. Statin drugs are prescribed to lower cholesterol; beta-blockers and clonidine are prescribed to lower blood pressure; and anti-diabetic drugs for diabetics. All of these drugs cause damage to CoQ10 levels in the body and depletes other nutrients such as beta-carotene, folate, calcium, magnesium, zinc, phosphate, and vitamins A, B12, D, E, and K. It is important that a CoQ10 supplement be dissolved in an oil to be fully absorbed in the body. Empty the dry powder from a capsule onto a tablespoon of extra virgin olive or flax oil. It has very little taste.

Vitamin B Complex contains the essential B Vitamins - B1, B2, B3, B5, B6, B9, B12, plus vitamins Biotin, Choline, and Inositol. Vitamin B Complex is needed for the proper functioning of almost every process in the body. Vitamin B complex should be taken as a powder in capsule form with vitamin C as well as vitamin E. Used together these vitamins have been shown to assist each other.

All vitamins should be taken in a dry powder form in a capsule and never in a hard tablet. Tablets cannot be absorbed in the body because they contain binders like glue which keeps them from breaking and being damaged in shipping.

Health and diet maintenance require understanding food, proper exercise, and vitamin supplements. Remember the goal is to *establish and make a habit* exercising and choosing foods that are nutritious and healthful.

Chapter Twenty

Choose Safe Cosmetics

WE HAVE DISCUSSED WHAT GOES INTO the body but the beauty products we use topically also are a concern. Our skin is our largest organ and we must protect it. Some beauty products contain carcinogens and endocrine disrupting chemicals that absorb through our skin and increase breast cancer risk. It is important to be conscious of the toxic chemicals that may be in the cosmetics and toiletries you use. Discover what products you can do without and avoid products with chemicals, better yet, use fewer products.

Fake Products

A recent investigative study ("To Catch a Fake") on 20/20 ABC News on June 13, 2014, showed how many of our daily skin and hair products have been counterfeited. Many of these products are from China and their manufacturers deliberately add carcinogenic material such as formaldehyde, lead, and mercury that are used as preservatives, and copper for skin tightening.

Unfortunately, the beauty industry is virtually unregulated in the U.S. and many toxic chemicals like phthalates and parabens (chemical preservatives used to lower costs) can be found in the most common makeup, shampoos, lotions, and other personal care products. Be wary of brand named products purchased for less money, particularly in discount stores. There is a reason they are cheap!

It is good to look for natural beauty products or make your own out of common household ingredients. For example, I use plain olive, avocado, coconut oil as a skin moisturizer for chapped and cracked hands. (See end of chapter for some easy homemade recipes for makeup and toiletries.)

Decrease the number of toxic chemicals that may be in the cosmetics and toiletries you use. Aluminum salts are used as the active antiperspirant agent in underarm cosmetics. This is especially important in relation to the breast because it is a local area of application. Aluminum clinical studies show a high incidence of breast cancer in the upper outer quadrant of the breast.[1] Find aluminum-free formula underarm antiperspirants if you don't wish to make your own. Aluminum has also been linked with Alzheimer disease. Reports have also suggested that underarm cosmetics products contain many harmful substances, which can be absorbed through the skin or enter the body through nicks caused by shaving. Some scientists have also proposed that ingredients other than aluminum in underarm antiperspirants or deodorants may be related to breast cancer because they are applied frequently to an area next to the breast.[2, 3] It is best to also stay clear of any beverage in aluminum cans. Individual brands aside, some products are just bad news.

Things to avoid:

- Anti-aging creams with alpha hydroxy acid (AHA, like glycolic acid or lactic acid) or beta hydroxy acid (BHA, as in salicylic acid)
- Hair dyes, especially dark permanent dyes
- Liquid hand soaps and antibacterial soaps with triclosan/triclocarban

- Nail polish and removers with formaldehyde, Dibutyl phthalate (DBP) which is a commonly used plasticizer, or toluene (a colorless, water-insoluble liquid with the smell associated with paint thinners which can be contaminated with benzene)
- Skin lighteners with hydroquinone (benzene)
- Heavily scented products
- Moisturizers, ointments, and skin creams with petroleum which can be contaminated with polycyclic aromatic hydrocarbon (PAH) (one of a class of chemical compounds which are pollutants)
- Fungicides, shaving creams, hair gels, and hair coloring containing nonylphenol
- Hair spray, gel, mousse, or shaving cream that contains isobutane, a propellant that can be contaminated with 1,3-butadiene
- Sunscreens with UV filters that mimic estrogen
- Toothpaste containing fluoride which can cause dental fluorosis from swallowing too much fluoride

Each cosmetic product you eliminate decreases the number and quantity of chemicals to which the body is exposed. Avoid synthetic fragrance, which can contain hundreds of chemicals, including toxic phthalates (a group of chemicals to soften and increase the flexibility, transparency, and longevity of plastic and vinyl are used in a wide range of common products that are easily released into the environment which can be inhaled). Opt for products that are fragrance-free or that contain natural fragrances like essential oils.

To find out whether your products are safe, visit Environmental Working Group's Skin Deep cosmetics safety database at, www.ewg.org. It has information for sun care, makeup, skin care, hair products, nail products, fragrance, oral care and men's products.

Label Reading

Read labels for specific information on a product's ingredients, rather than relying on advertising claims like "organic" or "natural." Look for USDA-certified organic labels on the packaging and/or product labels. If the product contains at least 70 percent <u>certified</u> organic content (excluding salt and water) AND is overseen by a certifying agent, the product qualifies for the "made with" organic labeling category. To qualify for the "organic" category and use the USDA organic seal, ingredients also need to be certified organic (this type of labeling is also used for food).[4] But a claim of "made with organic ingredients" or "made with natural ingredients" still leaves plenty of room for harmful synthetics.

Good ingredients are words that you've heard before, like aloe or lavender. Bad ingredients are words you can't even pronounce and are probably chemicals. Chemicals sound like chemicals. Avoid products with DMDM hydantoin and imidazolidinyl urea, (both derived from formaldehyde and used a preservatives). Parabens are rapidly absorbed and metabolized, and the excreted preservatives have been found in breast cancer tumors. Product with parabens or any word ending in "paraben", "PEG" compounds (polyethylene glycols), petroleum-based compounds that are widely used in cosmetics as thickeners, solvents, softeners, and moisture-carriers should be avoided. Lastly, stay away from products with words ending in "-eth", triclosan, triclocarban, triethanolamine (TEA), hydroquinone and oxybenzone. These all are toxic chemicals.

Dark Spot Correctors

Many dark spot correctors still use ingredients that have been proven dangerous. Using a product that contains hydroquinone and mercury as ingredients can cause serious damage to your health. Hydroquinone is a carcinogenic chemical banned in most countries except in the US. Besides increasing skin sensitivity, it has been linked to tumor growth. This is not something you want to be rubbing into your skin. Mercury can damage the kidneys and nervous system. It's used more often than you think, so always, <u>read</u> the label before buying!

For a dark spot corrector to be effective, it has to contain the right ingredients. Many correctors claim to be using the best, but be careful as many do not use the right amounts of ingredients to really get results.

Here are the proven ingredients to look for when buying dark spot remover/correctors:

- Alpha Arbutin: A compound derived from organic materials, Alpha Arbutin blocks the effects of melanin on the skin, removing dark spots quickly and safely.
- Resveratrol: Another powerful melanin blocker. This has been clinically shown to reduce melanin production by 50%.
- Sepicalm-S: This compound is one of the most powerful anti-pigment and anti-inflammatory agents on the market and is perfect for reducing acne scarring.

Choose Safe Nail Salons

Nail salons are known to be filled with chemicals. If you go for a manicure or pedicure, select a salon that stocks only nail polishes free of the toxic trio (formaldehyde, toluene—which can be contaminated with benzene—and dibutyl phthalate). Do not shave your legs before you receive a pedicure as it is a porthole for bacteria. Also look for a salon that has good ventilation for the entire shop, that the floors and all equipment are clean and disinfected to prevent fungus and that the technician wears gloves. Choosing a salon that engages in these safety practices can help protect your health and the health of the workers who are there every day. Make sure you can communicate with the nail technician. Miscommunication is a primary cause of nail salon infections and lawsuits from infections. A good salon makes you feel comfortable about the service that you are receiving.

How did a toxic poison end up in our water and toothpaste?

In 1945 local water treatment facilities began to add sodium fluoride to water supplies as a medical treatment for the sole purpose of preventing tooth decay (a non-waterborne disease). All other water treatment chemicals are added to improve water quality or safety, which fluoride does not do. Fluoride later crept into toothpaste as an ingredient for the prevention of tooth decay. Sodium fluoride in our water and toothpaste is not a pharmaceutical grade additive but rather an industrial waste by-product from aluminum manufacturing. Fluoride toothpastes make up more than 95% of all toothpaste sales. It is also interesting that toothpastes are classified as cosmetic products. The amount of fluoride contained in fluoride toothpaste should be indicated on the toothpaste tube, although this information may sometimes be hard to locate. It may appear after the label "Active ingredient" or as a component under "Ingredients" on the toothpaste tube.

Adding fluoride to our water supply and toothpaste created a multi-billion dollar industry and enabled manufacturers to sell this worthless toxic byproduct of aluminum to local municipalities for a profit.

The Center for Disease Control and Prevention states that dental fluorosis is a defect in tooth enamel caused by excessive fluoride intake during the tooth-forming years (age 0 to 8). In its mild forms, dental fluorosis presents as cloudy white splotches and streaks on the teeth, while in its moderate and severe forms, fluorosis can cause extensive brown and black staining along with pitting and crumbling of the enamel. Children who ingest a lot of fluoride toothpaste (whether accidentally or purposefully) can develop the disfiguring brown and black stains of advanced fluorosis, particularly if they also drink fluoridated water. Fluorosis on the front teeth, even in its "mild" forms, but especially in its severe forms, can cause self-esteem problems for a child, particularly when they reach adolescence. It is unfortunate however, that the CDC still promotes fluoridation.

No disease, not even tooth decay, is caused by a "fluoride deficiency."[5] Not a single biological process has been shown to require fluoride. On the contrary there is extensive evidence that fluoride can interfere with many important biological processes as well as with numerous enzymes.[6] In combination with aluminum, fluoride interferes with G-proteins.[7] Such interactions give aluminum-fluoride complexes the potential to interfere with growth hormones and in the processes of neurotransmission and intercellular signaling in the brain.[8] More and more studies indicate that fluoride can interfere with biochemistry in fundamental ways.

In 1977, Dean Burk, PhD, former head of the Cytochemistry Section at the National Cancer Institute and John Yiamouyiannis, PhD biochemist, conducted a study which compared ten largest U.S. cities with fluoridation and ten largest without. What researchers found was that following fluoridation, deaths from cancer went up immediately—in as little as a year. Skepticism of his claim led to a debate for years. The debate resurfaced in 1990 when a study by the National Toxicology Program, part of the National Institute of Environmental Health Sciences, performed a study that found rats who drank fluoridated water showed an increase in tumors and cancers in oral squamous cells, developed a rare form of bone cancer called osteosarcoma, showed an increased in thyroid follicular cell tumors and developed a rare form of liver cancer known as hepatocholangiocarcinoma.[9] However, other studies in humans and in animals have not shown an association between fluoridated water and cancer so there still is skepticism.

Once fluoride is put in the water it is impossible to control the dose each individual receives because people drink different amounts of water. Being able to control the dose a patient receives is critical. Some people (manual laborers, athletes, diabetics, and people with kidney disease) drink substantially more water than others.

The Arizona Republic and azcentral.com hosted a live online chat with experts on the issue of fluoridation voicing lengthy pros and cons from Will Humble, director of the Arizona Department of Health Services, and Deborah Dykema, a Phoenix-based osteopathic physician. Humble contended that fluoride helps prevent tooth decay and has no serious side effects. Dykema and opponents of fluoridation argued that Phoenix was putting residents at risk by providing a medicine in unlimited dosages introduced studies that linked fluoride to thyroid and neurological problems as well as a study performed by Harvard confirmed a direct inverse link between fluoridation of water and children's IQ. Children in fluoridated communities had a statistically significant lower IQ than children in non-fluoridated communities. The online debate was enough to sway the Phoenix residents. Since September 2012

168

the City of Phoenix, Arizona has stopped putting fluoride in its water supply after receiving a flood of comments from angry residents. Phoenix saved about $582,000 per year, or about 39 cents per resident, by ceasing to put fluoride in water.

Thank you Phoenix!

America, Wake Up!

Healing from cancer without chemotherapy and radiation has made me more diligent in what goes in my body as well as on it. Throughout my research I have learned how toxic we can become if we don't "wake-up" to how exposed we are to chemicals. For this reason I make my own cosmetics as much as possible with organic ingredients.

Choose Safe Cosmetics

Choose Safe Cosmetics

Fun Homemade Naturals

Thirty Minute Hand and Body Cream

- 1/2 cup coconut oil
- 1/2 cup shea butter
- 1/2 cup cocoa butter
- 3 tbsp beeswax
- 1/4 cup apricot kernel oil or almond oil
- 1 tsp vitamin E oil
- 1 tbsp aloe vera gel
- 5-10 drops essential oils: almond, orange or lavender
- 1 1/4 cup hot filtered water (it must be the same temperature of the oils or it will clump)

Heat the coconut oil, shea butter, cocoa butter, and beeswax over low heat until melted. Remove from heat and stir in liquid oils, essential oils, and aloe vera. While oils are cooling it turns darker in color and loses clarity (about 15 minutes) in a separate pan, heat water, but do not allow it to a boil. With a mixing wand, or in a blender, slowly add hot water to the melted oils and beeswax mixture until it is creamy and fluffy. Pour into two 4oz mason jars or containers of your choice and let cool.

Fifteen Minute Lip Balm

- 2 tbsp beeswax
- 2 tbsp shea, cocoa, or mango butter
- 2 tbsp coconut oil
- 20 drops of essential oil of choice (peppermint essential oil for a cooling and refreshing lip balm)

Put about an inch of water in the bottom of a small pan and turn on medium heat. Place a half pint size jar (8 oz mason jar) in the water. Do not get water inside the jar. Place all ingredients except the essential oils in jar and slowly melt to a liquid and remove pan from heat. Stir in the essential oils. Wrap the lip balm containers in a rubber band and stand them up right in another wider glass jar to keep them sturdy and steady while filling. Use a child's medicine syringe to quickly fill the containers. (The jar with the mixture should remain in the heated water to keep the ingredients liquid while filling the lip balm tubes.) The mixture will settle slightly as it cools. Top the containers after about two minutes as they start to harden. Let containers sit without touching them for several hours or until completely hardened. Store in a cool dry place (they will last for at least a year if stored correctly). This amount fills about 18 tubes. Tubes and syringe can be purchased online.

Homemade Eye Shadow

Eye shadow is probably the easiest thing to make at home. There are many natural ingredients that have color. Mix ½ ounce of the shade that you like and add arrowroot to make your desired color. Store it in a 1 oz container. (I have not found any acceptable healthy blue coloring)

- o Browns – cocoa powder, cinnamon, or nutmeg. Combine with arrowroot powder to make lighter.
- o Reds – beet root powder or hibiscus powder. Combine with arrowroot powder to make lighter.
- o Oranges/orange-reds – saffron for orange. Combine saffron and beet root powder. For orange-red combine with arrowroot powder to make lighter.
- o Greens – Spirulina combined with arrowroot powder for different shades. You can get Spirulina capsules for as low as $6. Just make sure the capsules can be cut open. Use a mortar and pestle to obtain a more fine Spirulina powder.
- o Black/Grey – Activated charcoal mixed with arrowroot powder. You can get 100 charcoal capsules for just $9 which can be found in most health food stores or online. Just make sure the capsules that you can be cut open.
- o Micas – for glitter and sparkle

Natural Homemade Foundation Powder

Use 1 tsp arrowroot powder for dark skin

and 1 tbsp arrowroot powder for light skin

In a small 1/2 or 1 oz container mix in cocoa powder, or ground cinnamon, or nutmeg until it reaches the desired tone. For more of a "compact" foundation, use 5 drops at a time of olive or almond oil until it reaches the desired texture. Then use a brush to apply foundation. Make sure to tap off excess before applying to the face.

Homemade Mascara

2 tsp coconut oil

4 tsp aloe vera gel

1 tsp beeswax pellets

1 – 2 capsules of activated charcoal (for

black) or cocoa powder (for brown)

1 clean mascara container

Put coconut oil, aloe vera gel, and beeswax in a small saucepan over low heat. Stir until beeswax is completely melted. Open one to two capsules of activated charcoal (depending on desired color) and pour into oil mixture. Stir until completely incorporated. Remove from heat. Using a child's medicine syringe, squeeze mixture into the mascara tube which can be purchased online.

Make up Remover

3 tbsp Olive Oil

3 tbsp almond oil

1 tsp vitamin E oil

Shake all ingredients vigorously and store in a 1 ounce container. Dip a cotton ball into container to remove makeup. Coconut oil alone is also excellent for removing makeup.

Homemade Dark Spot Remover

Lemon juice acts as an organic bleaching agent. Simply squeeze out some juice from a lemon onto a small dish. Dip a cotton ball in the lemon juice and apply it to the spot. Let it rest for about half an hour and rinse it off with cold water. Repeat this at least two times a day. It takes 2 months for you to see positive results. If you have sensitive skin, dilute the lemon juice with water, rose water or honey.

Toothpaste

6 tbsp coconut oil

6 tbsp baking soda

25 drops essential oil (eucalyptus, peppermint or grapefruit)

1 tsp Stevia for a sweetener

Whip it well using a mixing wand until it is fluffy and creamy; store in a small jar with a secure lid

Toothpaste for three brushings

1 tsp baking soda

1 drop peppermint or lemon essential oil

Add a few drops of water with all ingredients and mix in a bowl until the paste is formed to brush your teeth.

Sunburn Relief

Try using a leaf of an aloe plant. Snip off a leaf and cut it lengthwise and squeeze out the gel directly onto the skin or into a bowl. Then rub into the burned area.

Acne Help

Try adding 2 to 3 drops of tea tree oil to ½ cup warm water. Saturate a cotton ball and dab onto affected areas.

Deodorant Powder

Mix ¼ cup baking soda and ¼ cup arrowroot in a small container. Baking soda stops odor and arrowroot absorbs moisture. Corn starch can be used in lieu of arrowroot. Dip fingertips in container and rub the powder under the arm.

Liquid Deodorant

In a small spray bottle combine ¼ cup aloe vera gel, ¼ cup rubbing alcohol or witch hazel (these two kill bacteria-causing odors), and ¼ cup bottled or distilled water. For aroma add 10 drops antibacterial essential oil such as lavender, peppermint, orange, or sandalwood. Shake well to blend, spray on, and let dry.

I have not used store bought deodorant in over twenty years. I also use plain rubbing alcohol when I don't have time to make deodorant.

It's up to you to make the right choices.

Chapter Twenty-One

Cancer-Not the End

CANCER GAVE ME HEALTH. What I have written has taken four years and is my story how I defeated cancer without chemotherapy or radiation. In 2011 I was told I was going to die if I didn't do the "standard" recommendations to deal with my diagnosis. Instead I chose to educate myself and apply what I learned to be a chemotherapy and radiation-free cancer survivor. I do not profess to be a doctor or a scientist. I have explained in my way, what I have learned and understand and believe to be true about chemotherapy and radiation and why I did not do it. I continue to attend my conventional and holistic doctor's appointments and do cancer testing. I still become a bit nervous when it is time to review my test results because there is no guarantee that I will never have a cancer recurrence. But I have lived longer than what is "statistically" expected, I continue to be cancer free, and I will continue with my lifestyle knowing I have a better chance of staying cancer free than those who chose not to do a lifestyle change.

With the millions of dollars spent each year to fight the war on cancer, the medical community still has *not* found a cure. But it *is* known cancer cells differ from normal cells. A side effect that occurs months or years after traditional cancer treatment, patients can experience "long-term side effects". Many people who have received a chemotherapy cancer treatment have a risk of developing long-term side effects. Evaluating and treating these late effects are an important part of survivor care. Depending on the type of cancer diagnosis, maybe chemotherapy or radiation is not the correct answer for a cure.

- Fact: Chemotherapy drugs cause organ and tissue damage and other cancers
- Fact: Chemotherapy with radiation therapy magnifies organ and tissue damage and other cancer development; radiation alone can also cause other cancers
- Fact: Nutritional treatments and alternative treatments work well with conventional treatments. Oncologists should be encouraged to promote these alternatives rather than just introducing fear to the patient. There is no evidence that nutritional supplements interfere with traditional cancer treatments. In fact they enhance their effectiveness.

With these facts in mind, it is important for me to reiterate some important healthy changes to be incorporated in your new lifestyle to maintain your health or help you defeat cancer, diabetes, pancreatic or, any chronic diseases. Eating an alkalizing diet rich in flavonoids, vitamins and minerals balance the pH levels. It is a lifestyle high in fruits and especially vegetables.

Juicing is the best for a cancer protocol as it gives the cancer patient the nutrients that just *eating* fruit and vegetables cannot provide. It is important to start integrating juice into your new lifestyle daily. Once juicing is started keep juicing only if it is two 10 to 12oz vegetable juices a day. Vegetable juices are more important than fruit juices to improve the immune system as vegetable juicing reverses the effects of many degenerative illnesses. These changes take time and effort and do not come easily. It takes work to be and stay healthy.

There is no magic pill.

1   Get support and exercise even if only walking. Remember 60 minutes of daily exercise can be broken into two 30 minute increments.

2   Watch the scale. If you fall off your regular healthy lifestyle routine during a vacation or business trip, don't fret. Get back on course as soon as possible. Make it a learning experience, not a failure.

3   Eat breakfast every day as it sets the tone for the rest of your day.

4   Boost the immune system and take vitamin supplements. Avoid immune suppressing foods like omega 6 fats and sugar that stimulate cancer growth and add weight.

5   Choose safe cosmetics and watch out for fakes. What goes on our body is just as important as what goes into it. Our skin is our largest organ and we must protect it as well.

6   Be wary of fluoride. It is a poison. Tooth decay is not caused by a "fluoride deficiency."

7   Pay attention to produce and pesticides. Remember that genetically modified foods contain more pesticides. Strive for organic as much as possible.

8   All meat that is consumed should be organic grass fed, flax fed or wild game. Every beef eating American, for more than 50 years, has been exposed to steroids and growth hormones and now are additionally exposed to pesticide laden genetically modified crops that are fed to animals. Milk or beef cattle injected with growth hormones contain substantially higher amounts of potent cancer tumor promoting substances. Growth hormone laden milk or meat contains higher levels of pus, bacteria, and antibiotics.

It is my opinion utilizing nutritional treatments must be done by word of mouth and not within the traditional medical establishment because conventional medical doctors do not receive enough nutritional training to understand the powerful effects of proper nutrition. In many cases doctors can only prescribe treatments approved by the FDA. If they don't, they can be sued or lose their medical license if they administer an alternative cancer treatment.

The truth is that cancer can be prevented, controlled, and even most cancers can be cured through nutritional guidance, a positive attitude, and changes in lifestyle. It has been known for decades that *many* alternative medicines, including plant based foods and herbs, have positive and beneficial effects to reduce cancer growth. However, conventional medicine says nutrition cannot cure. It is my belief that in order to do so, the medical community must embrace nutrition and understand why and how nutrition works.

I want to help people to "Wake-Up" and make good lifestyle changes. But I can only help if people allow themselves to be helped. That is another reason I wanted to write this book. I want to share my knowledge of what I have learned and show people that change is possible and what happens when a change is implemented. You can live!

Three years ago I was concerned for my friend's life. It took a year for her to see the benefits of what I was doing. Living by example proves to be very beneficial when it comes to helping others. She was finally able convince her husband she needed to change her lifestyle and that it was *her* change, not his. She states it took awhile but when the change was truly put into practice, she started to gain weight without being hospitalized, and felt stronger, and her recovering from chemotherapy became easier. She thanked me for being there for her and helping her through tough times. She is my friend; I love her and I will continue to support her.

It is your right to know and be informed about all aspects of your diagnosis and treatments. It is ok to disagree with doctors, friends or relatives. They mean well and want to help, but after all, it's not their body.

Whatever decision you make, don't look back, and never say, "I wish I could have" or "I wish I should have". And don't regret your decision! No matter what choices I made, the bottom line is: It is up to you how you approach your health based on your circumstances and your research and your understanding.

I sincerely wish you all the best.

Select Bibliography

Charlotte Gerson: *Healing the Gerson Way, Defeating Cancer and Other Chronic Diseases* Obviously this book has had a positive impact on my life. It contains information a patient needs to utilize the Gerson Therapy. Additionally, it thoroughly details how the therapy works in the body and with many modern illnesses.

— *The Gerson Therapy: The Amazing Nutritional Program for Cancer and Other Illnesses* One of the first alternative cancer therapies, the Gerson Therapy has successfully treated thousands of patients for over 60 years and reveal the powerful healing effects of organic fruits and vegetables.

Charlotte Gerson and Morton Walker, D.P.M: *70 Years of Success! The Gerson Therapy The Proven Nutritional Program for Cancer and Other Illnesses.* This is a revised and updated edition of alternative medicine therapist Charlotte Gerson and medical journalist Morton Walker have collaborated to reveal the healing effects of organic fruits and vegetables. Not only can juicing reverse the effects of many degenerative illnesses-it can save lives.

Dr Max Gerson: *A Cancer Therapy: Results of Fifty Cases and the Cure of Advanced Cancer by Diet Therapy 6th Edition* Originally it was a reference for medical professionals and is a summary of thirty years of clinical experimentation. It is a Cancer therapy that explains the Gerson Therapy in detail and recounts 50 cases presented by Dr. Gerson. It is a medical dictionary of sorts and is very helpful for those on the Gerson Therapy.

David Servan-Schreiber, MD & PHD: *Anticancer: A New Way of Life* A remarkable story about a cancer survivor and scientist who changed his diet and lifestyle, learned to exercise regularly, manage stress and avoid contaminants in his body as best as possible. His research has led to the knowledge that a healthy immune system can keep the body's inflammation down which reduces cancer growth. The traditional Western diet is pro-inflammatory while a vegetarian diet, and Mediterranean diet as well as Indian and Asians cuisine are anti-inflammatory.

Suzanne Somers: *Breakthrough, Eight Steps to Wellness* Because of this book, I have learned the value of bioidentical hormone therapy and bioflavonoids. The book has a Q&A format with doctors who are curing cancer and using proven remedies and preventative care that most doctors just aren't talking about with patients. This book gave me HOPE and lead to much more.

Russell L. Blaylock, MD: *Natural Strategies for Cancer Patients* He is one of the doctors interviewed in Suzanne Somers: *Breakthrough, Eight Steps to Wellness*. His book is a must read to learn how to minimize the side effects of chemotherapy and radiation and increase the benefits of treatment programs to fortify the immune system and maintain strength and vitality. It explains which foods are uncommon cancer-fighting foods, which supplements can help and hurt, how certain fats and oils enhance the body and how flavonoids enhance the effectiveness of chemotherapy while adding a significant layer of protection to healthy cells.

— *Health and Nutrition Secrets that Can Save Your Life* Discover how chemicals such as mercury, fluoride, food additives, heavy metals, pesticides and herbicides are destroying our bodies. Find out what we encounter every day that can lead to unexpected health complications and life-threatening disorders.

William Davis, MD.: *Wheat Belly* The author is a cardiologist and medical director for Track Your Plaque, an online heart disease prevention program. Lose the wheat, lose the weight, and find your path back to health. Understand that today's wheat is genetically modified and learn about the good wheat: einkorn and emmer.

Richard Béliveau, Ph.D. and Dr. Denis Gingras: *Foods That Heal Cancer: Preventing Cancer Through Diet.* Richard Béliveau, leading biochemist, has teamed up with Denis Gingras, a French researcher in the Molecular Medicine Laboratory of UQAM-Hôpital Sainte-Justine, to describe the science of food and which properties of particular foods are the active cancer-fighting elements. They precisely explain how different foods work to protect the body against different cancers and show which foods will be most effective. By understanding the science behind these therapeutic benefits, they have proven why it is so critical to add these cancer fighting foods to our diet and how easily it can be done.

Harold W. Manner, PhD.: *The Death of Cancer* Dr. Manner is a professor of Biology and Chairman of the Biology Department of Chicago's Loyola University. His treatment is based in research which builds on a controversial theory of nutrition therapy can contain, prevent, and cure cancer using laetrile. His book is about a metabolic program that claims cancer can be treated by being controlled through nutritional guidance, a positive attitude, and changes in lifestyle.

Esther and Jerry Hicks: *The Law of Attraction* This book helped me in my healing process with cancer and is continually helping me in my daily life. Here is an excerpt from the book that says it all. "Learn about the omnipresent *Laws* that govern this Universe and how to make them work to your advantage. The understanding that you'll achieve by reading this book will take all the guesswork out of daily living. You'll finally understand just about everything that's happening in your own life as well as in the lives of those you're interacting with. This book will help you to joyously be, do, or have anything that you desire!"

Cherie Calbom and Maureen Keane: *Juicing for Life* This book showcases the benefits of fresh fruit and vegetable juicing, including what juices can help with certain ailments. It contains fresh, vitamin-rich fruit and vegetable juicing recipes that can help you lose weight and improve your health by boosting your metabolism and cleansing your entire body.

Theodore A. Baroody, MA, DC, ND, L.M.T., PhD (Nutrition): *Alkalize or Die* Dr Baroody's book discusses how excess acids in the small intestines can negatively affect that vital organ and how overall health can be achieved by balancing the acidity in the body. The book describes and gives understanding how alkalizing the body can boost overall health and the health of specific areas of the body.

Sally Fallon Morell and Mary G. Enig, Ph.D.: *Nourishing Traditions* Challenges politically correct nutrition and the diet "Dictorats" and includes information on how to prepare grains, health benefits of bone broths and enzyme-rich lacto-fermented foods.

— *Nourishing Broth* This book outlines the science behind broth's and their unique combination of amino acids, minerals and cartilage compounds. The book explains the benefits of fresh broth; healing of pain and inflammation, increased energy from better digestion, lessening of allergies and recovery from Crohn's disease. It explains how eating disorders are lowered because of the fully balanced nutritional broth program which lessens cravings that makes most diets fail. It outlines the diseases that bone broth can help heal such as osteoarthritis, osteoporosis, psoriasis, infectious disease, digestive disorders, and even some cancers.

Thomas Yarema, M.D., Daniel Rhoda, D.A.S. and Chef Johnny Brannigan: *Eat Taste Heal* Written by a medical doctor, a patient, and an acclaimed chef who utilizes humankind's most ancient system of healthy living. The book explores the field of holistic health and nutrition.

Marlo Morgan: *Mutant Message Down Under* A book about the simple truths of nature that can be applied in our modern society. It is an insight on how to get back in touch with nature, inner knowledge, inner guidance, and faith.

John Gunther: *Death Be Not Proud* An American journalist and author who is best known today for this book, a memoir about the death of his teenage son, Johnny Gunther, who was only seventeen years old when he died of a brain tumor. This is a deeply moving book about a father's memoir of a brave, intelligent, and spirited boy.

William Howard Hay MD: *Health Via Food* The author is a New York doctor and lecturer. This is his story of how he cured himself of Bright's disease which was unable to be cured using accepted medical methods of the time. Using alternative methods he came up with the concept of food combining (also known as the Hay diet). His concept was that certain foods require an acid pH environment in digestion, and other foods require an alkaline pH environment, and that both cannot take place at the same time, in the same environment.

Articles

http://cancerres.aacrjournals.org/content/68/21/8643.long   A History of Cancer Chemotherapy by Vincent T. DeVita, Jr. or Edward Chu, Yale Cancer Center, Yale University School of Medicine

http://aseh.net/teaching-research/teaching-unit-better-living-through-chemistry/historical-sources/lesson-2/Merrill-Food%20Safety%20Regulation-1997.pdf   Richard A Merrill: *Food Safety Regulation-Reforming the Delaney Clause* is a forty page research document that outlines the potential threats to food safety regulations, cosmetic safety, and the regulations of added carcinogens in food. It reflects a distrust of the administration of food and the hold the US Congress has retained for itself as the primary authority to decide not only how food "safety" should be pursued, but what food "safety" means.

http://www.jvascsurg.org/article/S0741-5214(10)01727-1/fulltext *The History of Radiation Use in Medicine* by Amy B Reed, MD at the Heart and Vascular Institute, Penn State Hershey College of Medicine, Hershey, PA

Website information

www.gerson.org The Gerson Therapy is a natural treatment that activates the body's extraordinary ability to heal itself through an organic, vegetarian diet, raw juices, coffee enemas, and natural supplements. The Gerson Institute is a non-profit organization in San Diego, California, dedicated to providing education and training in the Gerson Therapy, an alternative, non-toxic treatment for cancer and other chronic degenerative diseases.

www.longevitytlc.com The Longevity Center is a serious teaching facility where interested individuals can learn and experience the incredible healing power of nature, based on the brilliant work of Dr. Max Gerson who founded the Gerson Therapy. Dr. Donald Stillings, DC, the director of the Longevity Center, has been trained directly under Charlotte Gerson, the daughter of Dr. Max Gerson, at the Gerson Institute, graduating from the practitioner training in 2003. He holds multiple certificates from the Gerson Institute and was schooled in the mainstream clinical sciences. He followed that with graduate work in biochemistry, chemistry, and human physiology. Dr. Sillings' specialty is clinical nutrition and through his center I have learned the proper way to utilize food, supplements and the Gerson method of cancer healing.

www.burzynskiclinic.com The Burzynski Clinic was founded by Stanislaw R. Burzynski, M.D., PhD, cancer research and care has been inspired by the philosophy of the physician Hippocrates, *"First, do no harm."* The clinics treatments are based on the natural biochemical defence system of the body, which is capable of combating cancer with minimal impact on healthy cells.

www.foodmatters.tv People at Food Matters are committed to helping people help themselves. They believe that your body is worthy of good care. Think of them as your nutritional consultants to a healthier life. Check out the website for all kinds of health tips, the pros and cons when purchasing juicers, and information about healing clinics.

www.mercola.com This natural health website has health articles and food facts. If you go to http://articles.mercola.com/sites/Articledirectory.aspx you will see "Category" and under "Hot Topics" you can click on: "Aspartame, Cancer, Fluoride, Fructose/Sugar, GMO, Mercury Free Dentistry, Nutritional Typing, Vaccines, and Vitamin D".

www.dr-gonzalez.com Dr. Nicholas Gonzalez does nutritional approaches to cancer and other degenerative diseases. Click on "Case Reports" to learn about patients diagnosed with cancer who have responded to our nutritional/enzyme treatment.

www.breastcancerfund.org This organization aims to help expose and eliminate the environmental causes of breast cancer. Stop this disease before it starts.

www.preventcancer.com Here you will find the article "The American Cancer Society, More Interested in Accumulating Wealth than Saving Lives" written by Samuel S. Epstein, M.D., Chairman of the Cancer Prevention Coalition. Dr. Epstein has been active in publicizing claims on the carcinogenic properties of chlordane pesticides, growth hormones in milk, nitrosamines in bacon, saccharin, beverage preservatives, and other food additives. However, his work has attracted criticism from the U. S. Food and Drug Administration, which claimed that his book *The Safe Shopper's Bible* misleads consumers by labeling safe products as carcinogenic. He is a strong critic of the American Cancer Society.

www.ewg.org Environmental Working Group is a non-profit, non-partisan organization dedicated to protecting human health and the environment. Find out answers to burning questions: Do you know what's in your tap water? What about your shampoo? What's lurking in the cleaners underneath your sink? What pesticides are on your food? How about the farms, fracking wells, and factories in your local area? Do you know what safeguards they use to protect your water, soil, air, and your kids? Which large agribusinesses get your tax dollars and why? What are GMOs? What do they do to our land and water?

ww.cancer.gov/cancertopics/factsheet/Risk/BRCA. This website has a lot of information about cancer, BRCA1, BRCA2, and nutrition. However, it does focus primarily on chemotherapy and radiation cancer treatment. Nevertheless, it still offers a lot of valuable information.

www.cancer.org This site helped me learn and understand cancer. More than one million people in the United States get cancer each year. At this site you can find basic information about cancer, specific types of cancer, their risk factors, early detection, diagnosis, and treatment options.

www.russellblaylockmd.com I first learned about Dr. Russell Blaylock from Suzanne Somers: *Breakthrough, Eight Steps to Wellness.* Dr. Blaylock is a board certified neurosurgeon, author and lecturer and an expert on nutrition and toxins in food, cookware, teeth, and vaccines. His research discoveries have led to the idea that vaccines such as the H1N1 vaccine are dangerous or ineffective; that dental amalgams and fluoridated water are harmful to our health; and that aluminum cookware, aspartame, and MSG are toxic substances causing brain damage. Dr. Blaylock serves on the editorial staff of the Journal of the American Nutraceutical Association and is on the editorial staff of the Journal of American Physicians and Surgeons, official journal of the Association of American Physicians and Surgeons.

http://www.ams.usda.gov The U.S. Department of Agriculture's Agricultural Marketing Service administers programs that facilitate the efficient, fair marketing of U.S. agricultural products, including food, fiber, and specialty crops.

http://www.chrisbeatcancer.com At the age of 26 Chris Wark was diagnosed with stage III colon cancer in 2003. He had surgery, but refused chemotherapy. He is not a doctor but is an avid researcher on nutrition and natural therapies and he used nutrition and natural therapies to heal from cancer. He is alive and kicking, and cancer-free! It is wonderful site with all kinds of information about fluoride being a poison, cancer fighting food and natural therapies.

http://www.fluoridation.com   In depth views of fluoride poisoning and its effect on teeth, health, and the environment. The site also contains information about fraud, suppression, ethics and cover-ups.

http://fluoridealert.org/   More truth about fluoride regarding its poisoning attributes leading to death and brain damage and fifty reasons to oppose fluoridation.

http://www.naturalnews.com/002698_Ensure_food_marketing.html#ixzz2ycajO6c0   Nutritional values of Ensure

http://www.fakefoodwatch.com/2012/08/ensure-drink-sugary-fake-food-pseudo.html   Nutritional values of Ensure

http:// www.naturalhealthschool.com on-line nutrition self study course in herbals, nutrition, natural health, and pH balance

DVDs

Beautiful Truth is a documentary from filmmaker Steve Kroschel. It is about a 15 year old boy, Garrett, who was raised in Alaska on a wildlife reserve, tries to cope with the death of his mother. He falls into depression and nearly flunks out of school. Because of his father's concerns, he makes a decision to begin home-schooling Garrett. As his first assignment his father gives him the controversial book written by Dr. Max Gerson, a physician to claims that diet is capable of curing cancer. The boy sets out to research Dr. Gerson's therapy to find out if it is truly legitimate.

Cancer: The Forbidden Cures is a documentary film by Massimo Massucco exposes all the successful cures against cancer discovered in the last 100 years, and the reasons why they were suppressed. Cancer is the only disease that has been defeated dozens of times without anyone knowing it. In the last 100 years, dozens of doctors, scientists, and researchers have developed diverse and effective solutions against cancer only to be thwarted by the political and propaganda power of the drug-dominated medical profession. This is the story of Essiac, Hoxsey, Laetrile, Shark Cartilage, Mistletoe, and Bicarbonate of Soda all put together in a stunning overview that leaves no doubt that inexpensive cures for cancer do exist but are systematically blocked by Big Pharma because they come from nature and cannot be patented.

Dying to Have Known is a movie about filmmaker, Steve Kroschel's 52-day journey to find evidence to the effectiveness of the Gerson Therapy—a long-suppressed natural cancer cure which led him across both the Atlantic and the Pacific Oceans. He presents the testimonies of patients, scientists, surgeons and nutritionists who testify to the therapy's efficacy in curing cancer and other degenerative diseases, and presents the hard scientific proof to back up their claims. You will hear from a Japanese medical school professor who cured himself of liver cancer over 15 years ago, a lymphoma patient who was diagnosed as terminal over 50 years ago as well as noted critics of this world-renowned healing method who dismiss it out of hand as "pure quackery." So the question that remains is, "Why is this powerful curative therapy still suppressed, more than 75 years after it was clearly proven to cure degenerative disease?" The viewers are left to decide for themselves.

Food, Inc. is an important movie from filmmaker Robert Kenner, who exposes how America's food supply is now controlled by a handful of corporations the put profit ahead of consumer health, the livelihood of American farmers, the safety of workers, and the environment. It reveals the shocking truths of what we eat, how it is produced, and who we have become as a nation.

Food Matters is a film about America's current state of health. This feature-length documentary film from Producer-Directors James Colquhoun and Laurentine ten Bosch sets about uncovering the trillion dollar worldwide sickness industry and gives people some scientifically verifiable solutions for overcoming illness naturally. The focus of the film is in helping people rethink the belief fed to us by our modern medical and health care establishments. The interviews point out that not every problem requires costly, major medical attention and reveal many alternative therapies that can be more effective, more economical, less harmful and less invasive than conventional medical treatments.

Forks Over Knives by Lee Fulkerson and produced by John Corry is an American documentary film that advocates a low-fat, whole-food, plant-based diet as a way to avoid or reverse several chronic diseases and stresses that processed food should be avoided as well as food of animal origin.

Gerson Miracle examines many of the elements of the Gerson Therapy, explaining why we are so ill and how we have in our grasp the power to recover our health without expensive, toxic or mutilating treatments, using the restorative forces of our own immune systems. While the results seem miraculous, the real "miracle" lies within our own body and its healing processes. The documentary claims even the most advanced cases of cancer can be successfully reversed using this method which is NOT approved for use in the United States.

Second Opinion is a documentary by filmmaker, Eric Merola, about Ralph Moss, PhD who was Assistant Director of Public Affairs at Memorial Sloan-Kettering Cancer Center in New York City when he unveiled a cover-up of positive tests with America's most controversial anticancer agent, laetrile. He was ordered by Memorial Sloan-Kettering Cancer Center officials to falsify reports. He refused. Instead, he organized an underground employee group called Second Opinion to oppose this cover-up.

Reference Notes

Reference: Chapter 6 Proposed Chemotherapy and Radiation Treatments
1   American Cancer Society links radiation causing cancer: Retrieved from
    http://www.cancer.org/cancer/cancercauses/othercarcinogens/medicaltreatments/secondcancers
    causedbycancertreatment/second-cancers-caused-by-cancer-treatment-intro
2   Advances in radiation physics: refer to
    http://www.cancer.org/cancer/cancercauses/othercarcinogens/medicaltreatments/secondcancers
    causedbycancertreatment/index

Reference: Chapter 8 There Gerson Therapy, The Treatment
1   For added information visit Gerson Therapy: The Gerson Diet
    http://gerson.org/gerpress/the-gerson-therapy/
2   Charlotte Gerson quote refer to The Gerson Therapy: Detoxification
    http://gerson.org/gerpress/the-gerson-therapy/
3   John Gunther quote from his book *Death Be Not Proud* chapter 3 page 69 Recommended
    reading.

Reference: Chapter 10 The Importance of Testing on Monitoring Health
1   Dr. Samuel Epstein quote:http://articles.mercola.com/sites/articles/archive/2012/03/03/experts-
    say-avoid-mammograms.aspx
2   Non-bioidentical hormones: refer to: http://www.lifeextension.com/magazine/2009/10/
    bioidentical-hormones/page-01
3   Testosterone: refer to http://womensinternational.com/connections/testosterone.html

Reference: Chapter 12 Regulations and Manipulations
1   Counter Punch weekend edition August 14-16, 2009 (Monsanto's Man in the Obama
    Administration) www.counterpunch.org/2009/08/14/monsanto-s-man-in-the-obama-
    administration
2   The World According to Monsanto is a 2008 documentary film directed by Marie-Monique
    Robin Published on Apr 4, 2011 www.youtube.com/watch?v=aK7gAZS0lbY (a must see)
3   Organic Consumers www.organicconsumers.org/articles/article_18866.cfm
4   Richard A Merrill: Food Safety Regulation-Reforming the Delaney Clause:
    http://aseh.net/teaching-research/teaching-unit-better-living-through-chemistry/historical-
    sources/lesson-2/Merrill-Food%20Safety%20Regulation-1997.pdf
5   EBDCs (General Information) Mancozeb Fact Sheet http://pmep.cce.cornell.edu/profiles/
    fung-nemat/aceticacid-etridiazole/edbc/mancozeb-de-minimis.html
6   Federal Insecticide, Fungicide and Rodenticide Act, United States, December 2006:
    http://www.eoearth.org/view/article/152745/
7   Federal Food, Drug, and Cosmetic Act, United States, February 2007: http://www.eoearth.org/
    view/article/152744/
8   Consumer Reports "From Crops to Table" March 2015 Environmental Protection Agency.
    (n.d.). EPA's regulation of Bacillus thuringiensis (Bt) Crops [Webpage]. Retrieved from
    http://www.epa.gov/pesticides/biopesticides/pips/regofbtrops.htm.

9   Voice of America www.voanews.com/content/supreme-court-monsanto-soybeans-patents/1660356.html

10   Failure to Yield by Doug Gurian-Sherman of the Union of Concerned Scientists Tran-Pacific Partnership free-trade negotiation : http://www.ucsusa.org/assets/documents/food_and_agriculture/failure-to-yield.pdf

Reference: Chapter 13 Produce and Pesticides

1   Environmental Working Group http://www.ewg.org

2   Bienkowski, B. (2014, July 28). Songbirds dying from DDT in Michigan yards; Superfund site blamed: from the *Environmental Health News*.: www.environmentalhealthnews.org/ehs/news/2014/jul/dead-robins

3   Pesticides Tied to ADHD in Children in U.S. Study http://www.reuters.com/article/2010/05/17/us-adhd-pesticides-idUSTRE64G41R20100517

4   Pesticide Exposure in Children-Sources and Mechanisms of Exposure-Chronic Effects: http://pediatrics.aappublications.org/content/130/6/e1757

5   Mesnage, R., Defarge, N., de Vendomois, J.S. and Seralini, G-E. (2014). Major pesticides are more toxic to human cells than their declared active principles. *BioMed Research International 2014*. http://dx.doi.org/10.1155/2014/179691

6   "Dirty dozen" produce carries more pesticide residue, group says By Danielle Dellorto, Senior Medical Producer June 1, 2010: http://www.cnn.com/2010/HEALTH/06/01/dirty.dozen.produce.pesticide

7   Prevention-The Dark Side of Strawberries: http://www.prevention.com/food/healthy-eating-tips/strawberries-contain-large-amounts-chemicals-and-pesticides

8   A 'dangerous approach' to pesticides-Paul Helliker had a job for Dow Agro Sciences. http://www.theguardian.com/us-news/2014/nov/10/-sp-california-strawberry-industry-pesticides

9   Pesticide Action Network PAN-Chlorpyrifos http://www.panna.org/resources/chlorpyrifos#1

10   Lawsuit Urges EPA to Ban Neurotoxic Pesticide After 7 years of delays, groups call for action on chlorpyrifos http://earthjustice.org/news/press/2014/lawsuit-urges-epa-to-ban-neurotoxic-pesticide

11   9th Circ. Urged To Force EPA To Respond In Pesticide Row-Law360, New York http://www.law360.com/articles/576379/9th-circ-urged-to-force-epa-to-respond-in-pesticide-row

12   Oxford Journal accepted February 3, 2015 Human Reproduction: Fruit and vegetable intake and their pesticide residues in relation to semen quality among men from a fertility clinic: http://humrep.oxfordjournals.org/content/30/6/1342.full

13   Washington Post Pesticide Residue in Fruits and Vegetables Associated with Low Sperm Count http://www.washingtonpost.com/news/to-your-health/wp/2015/03/30/pesticide-residue-in-fruits-and-vegetables-associated-with-low-sperm-count/

14   European Union Bans Atrazine, While the United States Negotiates Continued Use by JENNIFER BETH SASS, PHD, AARON COLANGELO, JD: http://centerforhealthyhousing.org/Portals/0/Contents/Article0565.pdf

15   Organic Farming Research Foundation: http://www.ofrf.org/organic-faqs

16 Baker, B.P., C.M. Benbrook, E. Groth III, and K.L. Benbrook.2002 : http://www.ncbi.
    nlm.nih.gov/pubmed/12028642

Reference: Chapter 14 Not Eating Meat and Why
1   Richard A Merrill: Food Safety Regulation-Reforming the Delaney Clause
    http://aseh.net/teaching-research/teaching-unit-better-living-through-chemistry/
    historical-sources/lesson-2/Merrill-Food%20Safety%20Regulation-1997.pdf
2   Mother Earth News by Kim O'Donnell http://www.motherearthnews.com/real-food/food-
    policy/flexitarian-diet-zm0z14jjzmat.aspx
3   Pace Environmental Law Review by Sarah C. Wilson, "*Hogwash! Why Industrial Animal
    Agriculture is Not beyond the Scope of Clean Air Act Regulation*", 24 Pace Envtl. L. Rev. 439
    (2010) Available at: http://digitalcommons.pace.edu/pelr/vol24/iss2/5
4   National Resources Conservation Service-United States Department of Agriculture
    http://www.nrcs.usda.gov/wps/portal/nrcs/detail/mo/plantsanimals/?cid=stelprdb1042911
5   Organic Consumers: https://www.organicconsumers.org/scientific/growth-hormones-fed-beef-
    cattle-damage-human-health
6   Shirleys Welness Holistic Health for People and Animals; http://www.shirleys-wellness-
    cafe.com/NaturalFood/Bgh
7   Food and Drug Administration 2011 Summary Report on Antimicrobials Sold or distributed
    for Use in Food-Producing Animals: http://www.fda.gov/downloads/ForIndustry/
    UserFees/AnimalDrugUserFeeActADUFA/ucm277657.pdf
8   Food and Drug Administration 2010 Summary Report on Antimicrobials Sold or distributed
    for Use in Food-Producing Animals : http://www.fda.gov/downloads/ForIndustry/
    UserFees/AnimalDrugUserFeeActADUFA/UCM338170.pdf
9   Sustainable Table, Communications Foundation, Food Program rBGH:
    http://www.sustainabletable.org/797/rbgh
10 Antibiotics Used in Livestock Making us Sicker Than We Thought: September 11, 2013:
    http://civileats.com/2013/09/11/antibiotics-used-in-livestock-making-us-even-sicker-than-we-
    thought/
11 National Water Quality Inventory: Report to Congress 2004 Reporting Cycle submitted
    January 2009: http://water.epa.gov/lawsregs/guidance/cwa/305b/upload/2009_01_22_
    305b_2004report_2004_305Breport.pdf
12 Poultry and livestock exposure and cancer risk among farmers in the agricultural health study:
    http://www.ncbi.nlm.nih.gov/pubmed/22407136
13 Processed Meats Cause Cancer, October 26, 2015: http://www.npr.org/sections/thesalt/
    2015/10/26/451211964/bad-day-for-bacon-processed-red-meats-cause-cancer-says-who

Reference: Chapter 16 Knowledge is Important
1   Dr. Joseph Mercola: the Truth About a 40-Year Long Cover-Up of Laetrile Cancer Treatment
    http://www.secondopinionfilm.com/wp-content/uploads/2014/01/anatomy_
    of_a_coverup_so_02.pdf and
    http://articles.mercola.com/sites/articles/archive/2014/10/18/laetrile-cancer-research-cover-
    up.aspx#_edn15
2   US National Library of Medicine National Institutes of Health: "*Anti-tumor promoting effect of
    glycosides from Prunus persica seeds*": http://www.ncbi.nlm.nih.gov/pubmed/12576693

3   US National Library of Medicine National Institutes of Health: *"Amygdalin induces apoptosis through regulation of Bax and Bcl-2 expressions in human DU145 and LNCaP prostate cancer cells"* http://www.ncbi.nlm.nih.gov/pubmed/16880611

4   US National Library of Medicine National Institutes of Health: *"Amygdalin induces apoptosis in human cervical cancer cell line HeLa cells"*:
http://www.ncbi.nlm.nih.gov/pubmed/23137229

5   US National Library of Medicine National Institutes of Health: *"Amygdalin inhibits renal fibrosis in chronic kidney disease"* http://www.ncbi.nlm.nih.gov/pubmed/23525378

6   US National Library of Medicine National Institutes of Health: *"Amygdalin blocks bladder cancer cell growth in vitro by diminishing cyclin A and cdk2"*:
http://www.ncbi.nlm.nih.gov/pubmed/25136960

Reference: Chapter 17 Healthy Diets

1   David Servan-Schreiber, MD & PHD: *Anticancer: A New Way of Life* The traditional Western diet is pro-inflammatory and a vegetarian diet, Mediterranean diet, Indian and Asian cuisine are anti-inflammatory.

2   Dietary patterns and breast cancer risk: a systematic review and meta-analysis. *American Journal of Clinical Nutrition*: 2010 May; 91(5):1294-302. doi: 10.3945/ ajcn.2009.28796. Epub 2010 Mar 10. http://www.ncbi.nlm.nih.gov/pubmed/20219961 [PubMed Abstract]

3   Move over Mediterranean diet, the traditional Nordic diet could be key to losing weight *Independent News* September 2, 2014: http://www.independent.co.uk/life-style/food-and-drink/news/move-over-mediterranean-diet-the-traditional-nordic-diet-could-be-key-to-losing-weight-9706389.html

4   Say hello to the Nordic diet, a traditional Scandinavian style of eating by Gina Flaxman. *News.com.au*: August 4, 2014.http://www.news.com.au/lifestyle/health/say-hello-to-the-nordic-diet-a-traditional-scandinavian-style-of-eating/story-fneuzkvr-1227012485627

5   Healthy Habits in Norway by Jennifer Kahn: May 9, 2009: *Women's Health Magazine*:
http://www.womenshealthmag.com/food/healthy-lifestyle

6   *Olive Oil: Conditions of Competition between U.S. and Major Foreign Supplier Industries* (Inv. No. 332-537, USITC publication 4419, July 2013) is available on the USITC's Internet site at *http://www.usitc.gov/publications/332/pub4419.pdf*.

7   What is Real Olive Oil: http://realfoodforlife.com/which-olive-oil-to-buy-the-olive-oil-fraud

8   Tests indicate that imported "extra virgin" olive oil often fails international and USDA standards - UC Davis Olive Center, July 2010 http://olivecenter.ucdavis.edu/research/files/oliveoilfinal071410updated.pdf

Reference: Chapter 20 Choose Safe Cosmetics

1   Darbre PD. Aluminium, antiperspirants and breast cancer. *Journal of Inorganic Biochemistry* 2005; 99(9):1912–1919. [PubMed Abstract]

2   Darbre PD. Underarm cosmetics and breast cancer. *Journal of Applied Toxicology* 2003; 23(2):89–95. [PubMed Abstract]

3   Harvey PW. Parabens, oestrogenicity, underarm cosmetics and breast cancer: a perspective on a hypothesis. *Journal of Applied Toxicology* 2003 Sep-Oct; 23(5):285-8. [PubMed Abstract]

4   Agricultural Marketing Service of USDA and click on National Organic Program http://www.ams.usda.gov/

5   NRC 1993; Institute of Medicine 1997, NRC 2006

6   Waldbott George L, MD, 1998, *Fluoride*, 31:1, 13-20: The Preskeletal Phase of Chronic
    Fluoride Intoxication

7   J.Bigay *EMBO Journal*. 1987 Oct; 6(10): 2907–2913. PMCID: PMC553725
    Fluoride complexes of aluminum or beryllium act on G-proteins as reversibly bound analogues
    of the gamma phosphate of GTP. [NCBI Abstract]

8   Aluminofluoride complexes: new phosphate analogues for laboratory investigations and
    potential danger for living organisms. by Anna Strunecká & JiřÃ Patočka

9   FLUORIDATION-LINKED HUMAN CANCER BASED ON TIME-TREND MORTALITY
    DATA, By Dean Burk, Ph.D., U.S. National Cancer Institute, Retired, and Dean Burk
    Foundation, Inc., and John Yiamouyiannis, Ph.D., National Health Federation.(Abstract of
    paper presented at the Seventh Annual Conference of the International Society for Fluoride
    Research held at Zandervoort, Holland, February 8-10, 1976.)

Made in the USA
San Bernardino, CA
21 April 2016